Ultrasound–Guided Procedures and Investigations

Ultrasound–Guided Procedures and Investigations

A Manual for the Clinician

edited by

Armin Ernst
Beth Israel Deaconess Medical Center
Boston, Massachusetts, U.S.A.

David J. Feller–Kopman
Beth Israel Deaconess Medical Center
Boston, Massachusetts, U.S.A.

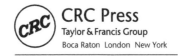

CRC Press
Taylor & Francis Group
Boca Raton London New York

CRC Press is an imprint of the
Taylor & Francis Group, an **informa** business

A TAYLOR & FRANCIS BOOK

First published 2006 by Taylor & Francis

Published 1991 by CRC Press
Taylor & Francis Group
6000 Broken Sound Parkway NW, Suite 300
Boca Raton, FL 33487-2742

© 2006 by Taylor & Francis Group, LLC
CRC Press is an imprint of Taylor & Francis Group, an Informa business

First issued in paperback 2019

No claim to original U.S. Government works

ISBN-13: 978-0-367-45401-2 (pbk)
ISBN-13: 978-0-8247-2921-9 (hbk)

Visit the Taylor & Francis Web site at
http://www.taylorandfrancis.com

and the CRC Press Web site at
http://www.crcpress.com

Library of Congress Cataloging-in-Publication Data

Catalog record is available from the Library of Congress

Preface

In the last few years, ultrasonography has become increasingly recognized as a helpful tool for the evaluation and management of patients in the intensive care unit, emergency department, and the operating room, as well as general hospital wards and outpatient clinics. Ultrasound guidance in thoracentesis and central venous catheterization is becoming the standard of care, and use of ultrasonography has significantly expedited the initial evaluation of the trauma patient. With the development of affordable and portable devices, ultrasound examinations are increasingly performed by nonradiologists.

This book is intended to serve as a resource for internists, pulmonologists, critical care physicians, surgeons, emergence medicine physicians, and anesthesiologists, as well as physicians in training. The chapters have been organized to provide a background in physics and imaging technology, review the literature pertinent to the most commonly performed procedures and nonprocedural applications of ultrasonography, and provide guidance on how to perform those examinations and procedures.

It is our hope that this book will inspire nonradiologists to become familiar with ultrasound and begin to use it as a tool in daily clinical practice in order to enhance patient care.

Armin Ernst
David Feller-Kopman

Contents

Contributors

Martin J. K. Blomley   Imaging Sciences Department, Imperial College, Hammersmith Hospital, London, U.K.

David O. Cosgrove   Imaging Sciences Department, Imperial College, Hammersmith Hospital, London, U.K.

Peter Doelken   Division of Pulmonary and Critical Care Medicine, Allergy and Clinical Immunology Medical University of South Carolina, Charleston, South Carolina, U.S.A.

Armin Ernst   Beth Israel Deaconess Medical Center, Boston, Massachusetts, U.S.A.

David Feller-Kopman   Medical Procedure Service, Interventional Pulmonology, Beth Israel Deaconess Medical Center, Boston, Massachusetts, U.S.A. and Harvard Medical School, Boston, Massachusetts, U.S.A.

James F. Greenleaf   Department of Physiology and Biomedical Engineering, Mayo Clinic College of Medicine, Rochester, Minnesota, U.S.A.

Christopher J. Harvey   Imaging Sciences Department, Imperial College, Hammersmith Hospital, London, U.K.

F. J. F. Herth   Department of Pneumology and Critical Care Medicine, Thoraxklinik, University of Heidelberg, Heidelberg, Germany

William Lunn   Interventional Pulmonary, Baylor College of Medicine, Houston, Texas, U.S.A.

Paul Mayo   Pulmonary and Critical Care Medicine, Beth Israel Medical Center, New York, New York, U.S.A.

Chris Moore   Department of Surgery, Section of Emergency Medicine, Yale University School of Medicine, New Haven, Connecticut, U.S.A.

Carlo L. Rosen   Beth Israel Deaconess Medical Center, Harvard Affiliated Emergency Medicine Residency, Boston, Massachusetts, U.S.A. and Harvard Medical School, Boston, Massachusetts, U.S.A.

Michael J. Simoff   Interventional Pulmonology and Bronchoscopy Services, Henry Ford Medical Center, Detroit, Michigan, U.S.A.

Carrie D. Tibbles   Beth Israel Deaconess Medical Center, Harvard Affiliated Emergency Medicine Residency, Boston, Massachusetts, U.S.A.

Jason A. Tracy   Beth Israel Deaconess Medical Center, Harvard Affiliated Emergency Medicine Residency, Boston, Massachusetts, U.S.A.

Momen M. Wahidi   Interventional Pulmonology, Division of Pulmonary and Critical Care Medicine, Department of Medicine, Duke University Medical Center, Durham, North Carolina, U.S.A.

1

ABCs of Ultrasound Imaging

James F. Greenleaf
Department of Physiology and Biomedical Engineering, Mayo Clinic College of Medicine, Rochester, Minnesota, U.S.A.

INTRODUCTION

"Imaging" is a term applied to the graphic depiction of an attribute, usually physical, and usually in a two-dimensional format. "Medical imaging" usually refers to procedures that produce attribute images of tissues within the body.

Ultrasonography has had an increasing role in medical imaging over the past 20 years. Its use continues to expand because of the availability of real-time imaging and Doppler blood flow measurement, new transducer design, better signal processing, miniaturization and computerization of electronics, elimination of X-ray radiation exposure, and high information versus cost ratios of the images.

Cardiology, obstetrics, gynecology, and other areas of medicine have been greatly impacted by ultrasound (US) imaging technology.

The tissues of the body can be divided broadly into two types, soft and hard. In general, US is used to image the soft tissues (1); however, some imaging of hard tissues, such as bone, has been reported (2). There are two main reasons for medical imaging, detection and diagnosis of disease. Disease is detected and/or diagnosed by evaluating changes in US images, relative to images from normal individuals or relative to previous images in the same individual.

To make a US image, local variations in some acoustic property, usually backscatter are detected using ultrasonic energy and are mapped into a two-dimensional format (3). This requires localization of the energy in depth and azimuth, using appropriate spatial and temporal control of the energy. This chapter describes: (i) the elements of US medical imaging, (ii) an example of an imaging system, (iii) energy transduction, (iv) beam control, (v) signal processing, and (vi) display methods.

ELEMENTS OF ULTRASOUND IMAGING

Images are formed by sending a short pulse of high frequency sound (2–20 MHz) into the body and detecting weak reflections from scatterers within soft tissues. The method is similar to radar or sonar but on a different scale. Images of these echoes and their positions within two-dimensional planes are called B-scans and exhibit highly detailed representations of the internal structures. The speed of sound (c) in tissue (c_t) (approximately 1500 m/sec) allows approximately 100 to 200 echo lines to be obtained and displayed in the time of a television frame (1/30 sec); thus the method can produce real-time images of the internal organs and tissues of the body.

Ultrasonic waves are produced with a ceramic that changes dimensions when subjected to an electric field. Axial, lateral, and transverse localization of the ultrasonic beam must be accomplished to successfully image two- or three-dimensional distributions of scatterers within a volume of tissue.

Axial Localization

Axial localization of the energy is done with short pulses of ultrasonic energy propagating through the tissue, which reflect from scatterers distributed throughout the volume. The time of arrival of the reflected pulse encodes the spatial position of the pulse if the speed is known.

Ultrasonic Wave Speed

Speed in the soft tissues of the body is assumed to be approximately 1540 m/sec in modern imaging instruments. This assumption is violated in many cases; for instance, the speed of sound in fat can be as low as 1430 m/sec (4). Because the speed is not known exactly, errors can occur in the imaging system depending on how disparate the various tissue speeds are. For instance, fat layers within or overlying tissues of interest can cause aberrations in the image because the ultrasonic wave propagation speed in fat is very low.

Velocity/Timing

The depth (z) from which a pulse returns is determined from the speed of sound (c) and the travel time (t) to and from the scatterer; i.e., $z = c \times t/2$.

Axial Resolution

The axial resolution of the US imaging system depends on the spatial length of the pulse, which is inversely proportional to the frequency bandwidth (Δf) of the pulse (Fig. 1). The spatial length of the propagating pulse determines the distance between consecutive scatterers that can be delineated in the image, and is thus called the axial resolution. A term

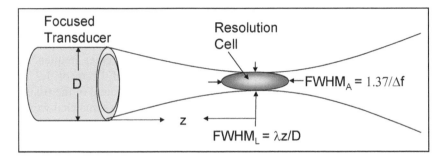

Figure 1
The resolution cell is the smallest volume from which the signal is received at one point in time. It depends on the aperture (*D*), the band width (Δf), the speed of sound (*c*), and the distance to the transducer (*z*).

used to define the resolution is full width half maximum amplitude (FWHMA), which refers to the width at half the peak amplitude of the envelope in the axial direction of the pulse of pressure traveling in the tissue. The relationship is:

$$FWHM_A = \frac{1.37 \, \text{mm} \, \text{MHz}}{\Delta F} \tag{1}$$

Imaging can be improved by ensuring that the pulse has low side-lobes in the time dimension. This can be done by providing pulses that have smooth Fourier transforms, ensuring a smooth time domain response (5).

Lateral Localization

Lateral localization of the focusing ultrasonic beam is accomplished by electronically controlling the phase and amplitude of the motion of the transducer surface in transmit mode and by dynamic focusing in receive mode. Most systems localize the transmit energy and the receive mode sensitivity to a line collinear with the transmit direction. Each line of sensitivity, or imaging beam, is transmitted, the echoes are received, and then a new line is incrementally scanned in the imaging plane. This procedure is repeated, scanning quickly within a plane to produce data for real-time backscatter imaging in the plane. Sometimes several adjacent receive lines are computed by the scanner in the beam forming section for each transmit. This increases the line rate and, thus, the frame rate.

Lateral resolution depends on the size of the aperture (*D*), the distance (*z*) from the surface of the transducer to the imaged point, and the effective wavelength ($\lambda = c/F$) of the pressure wave. The relationship is (6):

$$FWHM_L = \frac{\lambda z}{D} \tag{2}$$

This relationship gives the best-case resolution, stating that the larger the aperture (diameter or length of the transducer probe) in wavelengths, the better the resolution. Most medical transducer probes are approximately 2.5 cm across and typically run at center frequencies of 3.5 to 7.0 MHz, giving a resolution at a depth of 10 cm of 1.7 to 0.85 mm at best. Because of variations in the speed of sound in the tissue, some defocusing occurs, limiting the resolution to values somewhat worse than those estimated with Equation 2 (7).

Aperture Shading for Enhanced Contrast

An important aspect of medical imaging that is not important in nondestructive evaluation or other acoustic imaging disciplines is the contrast of the image. Contrast refers to the ability to image holes or regions of low scatter buried within regions of high scatter. Imaging with high contrast is desired because it produces images with very dark cysts and vessel lumens. This requires that the lateral and axial responses of the system have low side lobes.

High side lobes smear energy into the dark regions of the image, decreasing contrast. It is well known that the lateral field response of a square aperture is a sine function, which has high side lobes. Shading of apertures refers to changing the amplitude of the pressure over the surface of the imaging probe to decrease the side lobes. The lowest side lobes can be produced with Gaussian-like shading across the face of the probe. Many commercial medical imaging instruments shade the amplitude of the US signal over the aperture of the probe, in addition to tailoring the amplitude of the pulse in time to obtain the lowest side lobes possible in both the lateral and the axial directions.

Transverse Localization

Transverse localization refers to the control of the direction of the beam in the direction transverse to the scanning plane. Beam control is usually accomplished in this direction with physical acoustics. Lenses or other geometric methods such as curving the transducer are used to control the beam in the transverse direction. Of course, the beam is only focused at one range; thus the thickness of the resolution cell varies with depth from the transducer. This fact is often ignored when resolution is quoted for many commercial systems because only the lateral resolution is mentioned at the depth of transverse focus. The equation for the best achievable resolution in the transverse direction is the same as for the lateral resolution:

$$FWHM_T = \frac{\lambda z}{H}, \tag{3}$$

where H is the height of the transducer in the transverse direction. Some recent scanners focus electronically in the transverse direction using what are called 2.5-dimensional arrays. This means that the array is segmented in the lateral direction so that phased focusing is possible in that direction.

Resolution Cell

The resolution cell of the imaging system is defined as the volume of tissue that is within the lateral, axial, and transverse resolutions of the system. This represents the smallest physical domain from which information is acquired by the system for each point in time.

IMAGE ACQUISITION

The image is formed by transmitting energy in as narrow a beam as possible and recording the received echoes from the insonified pencil-like cylinder of tissue. The transducer then moves the beam and repeats the process. The ensemble of data from all beams is then assembled into an image. The process requires two parts, beam forming and beam scanning.

Beam Forming

Beams are formed in two ways, physically or electronically. Physical beam forming is done with lenses or with curved transducer elements. Electronic beam forming is done in transmit mode by phased pulsing of the elements of an array to produce a beam focused at some selected depth. Electronic beam forming in receive mode is done with the echo signals received on the array elements. Each signal is individually amplified, delayed, and summed to produce the selected receive beam.

Beam Scanning

The resulting beams are scanned physically or electronically. Physical scanning consists of translation or rotation of the transducer while launching the transmit beam and receiving echoes from the many different directions required to make up a two-dimensional image with electronic scanning. The beam can be launched or received in different directions with electronic phasing. The advantages of electronic phasing are speed and mechanical reliability. A disadvantage is the cost involved. For three-dimensional imaging, two approaches are used. The simplest is to mechanically translate an array, thus acquiring two-dimensional images through a volume. The other approach uses a two-dimensional array that can focus in a three-dimensional space, thus obtaining the data required to construct a three-dimensional image.

SYSTEM DESCRIPTION

The elements of an ultrasonic medical imaging system are shown schematically in Figure 2. The principle elements of the system, listed below, are discussed more fully subsequently:

Transduction: The electronic transmit pulse is converted to pressure waves that propagate into the tissue. The reflected pressure waves are

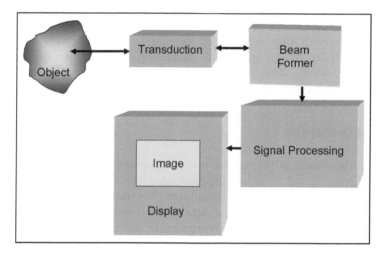

Figure 2
The principle components of the imaging system are the transducer, the beam former, the signal processor, and the display.

converted into an electronic signal in this extremely important element of the system.

Beam former: The ultrasonic beam is formed for both transmit and receive modes. This is done in many innovative ways comprising two general forms, physical acoustics and electronic phasing (described previously).

Signal processing: The received signal is processed to obtain images of scatterers or Doppler frequency shifts. Speed, attenuation, and other properties of tissue must be accounted for or measured. A great deal of postprocessing is now done to remove speckle, compound images, and knit several images together.

Display: The presentation of information to the user must be logical and consistent. The geometry of the beam distribution must be mapped into that of the viewing system.

Recording: Both static and dynamic recording are provided for the output images of the system and subsequent archival storage. In some systems, the raw data are stored so that a wide range of images can be reprocessed and displayed to the viewing physician after the patient has left the premises.

Transduction

A key part of the imaging system is the transducer. It must convert a voltage pulse of up to hundreds of volts into a pressure pulse and, within microseconds, be prepared to receive weak echoes producing a few microvolts of signal.

Transduction of the energy from electrical to mechanical in transmit mode and from mechanical to electrical in receive mode is universally done with the same transducer in medical imaging instruments. Most of the transducer materials used in current instruments are some form of lead zirconium titanate (8). Although the transducer is probably the most important element of the system, most of the expertise in making transducers remains an art.

Transducer Material

The transducer materials must be efficient electromechanical energy converters. This means that their electromechanical coupling coefficient for the thickness mode (K_t) must be as large as possible. However, because transducers are placed directly on the tissue, they must have the appropriate acoustic impedance to couple energy efficiently into the tissue. The impedance of tissue is approximately 1.5 Mrayl, but the impedance of typical transducers is approximately 33 MRayl. Impedance coupling is accomplished with electronic matching circuits and with physical matching layers on the front or back of the transducer. Transducers also must couple their energy efficiently into the transmission line that attaches them to the scanning machine. This requires that the dielectric coefficient (ε^S) be adjustable to fit the requirements of the specific array geometry. Of course the electrical and mechanical losses must be low, requiring $\tan \delta < 10\%$ (9).

Lead Zirconate-Titanate

Ceramics such as lead zirconate-titanate, modified lead titanate, and lead metaniobate are the most commonly used transducer materials. They have electromechanical values of $K_t = 40$–50%, $\varepsilon^S = 100$–2400, $\tan \varepsilon \leq 3\%$, and $Q_m > 50$.

Solid Phase

Some systems use solid phase ceramics cut into arrays or discs. The disadvantage of solid phase ceramics is that their impedance is 20 to 30 MRayl, too high to match tissues efficiently, even those with matching layers. A new method of reducing the acoustic impedance of ceramics is to use piezo-composites, which result in transducers with acoustic impedances closer to that of the tissues without altering the other electromechanical parameters.

Composite

Composites or piezo-composites are produced by kerfing the solid phase material as shown in Figure 3. The electromechanical values of these transducers are typically $K_t = 75\%$ and ε^S approximately 20–1000, with low losses. These materials are also physically flexible, allowing their use in complicated geometries (8).

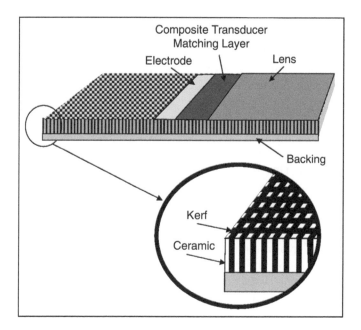

Figure 3
Composite transducers are made from solid phase transducers by dicing with a
saw and backfilling the kerfs with a polymer. The resulting transducer has low
impedance and a high coupling constant, in addition to physical flexibility.

Transducer Geometry and Beam Control

The principle geometries used in medical transducers are rectangular
(linear arrays) and circular. The circular geometry is usually physically
scanned and the linear array is electronically phased to produce a scan.

Disc

The simplest geometry for a transducer is a disc. When combined with a
lens or when shaped as a spherical cap, the disc geometry can focus in
both the lateral and transverse directions.

Single discs (Fig. 4) can be either single phase or composite.
They require only one signal channel but can focus with a lens at
only one depth. They are the least expensive transducers and can be
found on some of the inexpensive scanners. They are also used at
very high frequencies because cutting into annular or other geometries is difficult for very small transducers. Scanning with disc
transducers is accomplished with mechanical motion, either linear or
rotary.

Annular arrays are used to provide adjustable focus over a
long depth of field (Fig. 4). Phasing of the transmit signals on the
rings can focus the transmit signal at a selected depth. Delaying
the received signals with variable delay lines prior to summing the

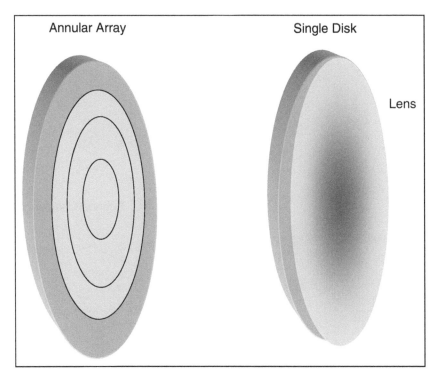

Figure 4
Comparison of annular and solid phase disc transducers. The annular array can
be dynamically focused in receive mode by changing the delay of the signals
from the different annuli prior to summing.

signals is done to sequentially change the receive focus, as the signals
echo from deeper and deeper in the tissue. The advantage of annular
arrays over linear arrays is that they have good transverse focus
throughout the depth of field. A disadvantage of annular arrays is
that they have to be mechanically scanned to obtain a two-dimensional
image.

Linear

The advantage of linear arrays is that they can be electronically phased to
produce beams that sweep out a rectangular two-dimensional plane
(Fig. 5). These arrays require no moving parts and provide potentially
high frame rates. A disadvantage is that they must be focused in the
transverse direction with physical acoustics using a lens or curved surface.
The result is a beam thickness that changes the transverse dimension with
depth.

One-dimensional arrays are also used to produce a fan- or sector-
shaped scanned region. Sector geometry for scanning is usually used
for cardiac imaging because the beam must image the heart using

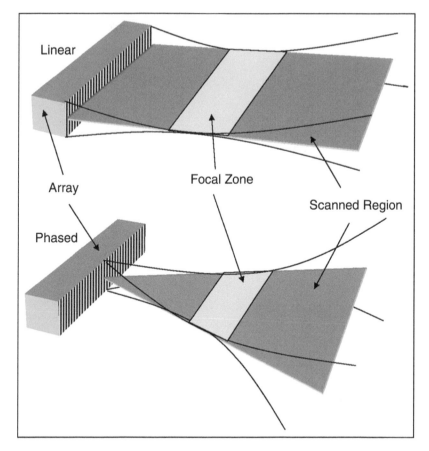

Figure 5
Arrays are used to produce two types of scans, the so-called linear scan
and the sector scan. Transverse focusing in the plane is done in transmit
by appropriately delaying the pulses to the elements. In receive, the focusing
is done with dynamic variable delay of the received signals on each of the
elements. The transverse focus is done with physical acoustics, lenses or
curvature.

the acoustic window between the ribs (Fig. 5). The disadvantage of
sector scanning is that interpolation of the beam signals received over a
triangular sector onto a rectangular TV raster is complicated.

Two-dimensional arrays are not yet widely used but may provide
control of the plane being imaged. They may also allow very fast acquisition
of data within a three-dimensional volume of tissue. The ability to focus
in both lateral and transverse directions may also be of benefit (Fig. 6).
Presumably, two-dimensional arrays can acquire three-dimensional data
very quickly. The disadvantage of two-dimensional arrays is that the
number of channels is very much greater than for one dimensional
arrays and the appropriate electronics for so many channels are very
expensive.

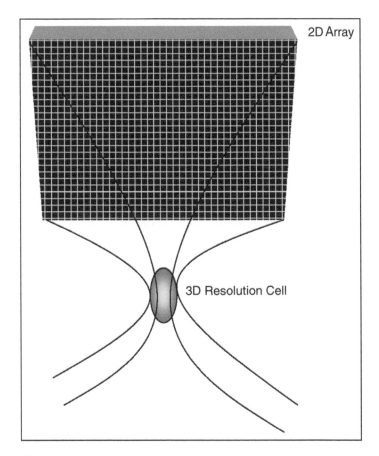

Figure 6
Two-dimensional arrays can focus in three dimensions. This allows volumetric imaging to be done without moving the array. Beam forming is done in a manner similar to that of the linear array but in two dimensions.

SIGNAL PROCESSING

The signal received from the transducer is not useful for display because it is radio frequency (RF) and must be turned into a non-negative magnitude to be displayed. In addition, attenuation and speed of tissue alter the signal and must be accounted for prior to imaging.

Attenuation Correction

Tissue is a low-pass filter. As the signal travels into the tissue, high-frequency components are absorbed more than low-frequency components, because the absorption coefficient of tissue is proportional to the frequency. Thus,

$$P(z) = P_0 e^{-\alpha z} \tag{1}$$

where $P(z)$ is pressure in the tissue and z is distance into the tissue along the propagating ultrasound wave, and where $\alpha \simeq 0.7$ and $n \simeq 1.2$ (10). Thus, two effects, the loss of amplitude and the loss of high frequency signal components with depth, must be corrected. The effects are corrected with a time variable gain (tvg) and a time variable filter circuit (tvf).

Time Variable Gain

The loss in amplitude, indicated by Equation 1, is usually corrected by amplifying the signal proportional to the depth from which the echo came. This amplifier is often manually controlled by the operator of the instrument, who sets the gain for various depths of the tissue to make the overall image look "flat" in amplitude.

Time Variable Filter

The time variable filter increases the gain for high frequencies as the signal comes from deeper in the tissue. This must be done carefully because noise can be enhanced but, generally, the image is improved.

Speed Assumptions

Most medical scanners use a fixed speed as the tissue speed. This is usually not variable and is fixed approximately 1540 m/sec.

Detection/Compression

The signal is usually full wave detected and low-pass filtered prior to being compressed for display. The magnitude signal is compressed because of the very high dynamic range of the signals (some 60–90 dB). Much of the information is in the low-level signals. For instance, the scatter within a fluid-filled cyst can determine whether it contains pure fluid or some possibly malignant cells or tissues.

Doppler Detection

Acoustic energy can be used to detect motion through the Doppler effect. The principle target for Doppler detection is density variations in the concentration of blood cells. Although their scattering strength is some two or three orders of magnitude lower than that of tissue, virtually all medical imaging systems now contain Doppler capabilities for detecting blood flow velocity. There are two general types of Doppler signals, C.W. and Pulsed, and there are two general types of signal analysis, frequency domain and time domain. All Doppler systems measure the ratio of the inner product of the reflector velocity $\vec{v}$ and the beam direction $\vec{k}$, to the speed of sound in the material (c), that is the Doppler shift (f_D) is (11):

$$f_D = f \frac{2\vec{v} \cdot \vec{k}}{c} \tag{2}$$

where f is the signal frequency and $\cdot$ is the inner product. Thus, the direction of the beam and the direction of the flow must always be known, if quantitative measurements are to be made.

The simplest type of Doppler device is the continuous wave system. The transmitter emits a continuous wave signal, which is received by a separate receiver. The received signal is mixed with the transmitted signal and the resulting tone (f_D, usually audible) is used to estimate the speed of the reflectors along the beam of the acoustic energy. In vessels, the sound varies greatly because of the pulsatile nature of the blood flow. However, trained operators can determine turbulence of the flow, patency of vessels, pulsatility indexes, presence of stenoses, and other characteristics of importance to vascular or cardiac specialists.

The advantage of the continuous wave method is that sampling is not a problem and aliasing does not occur, but the disadvantage is that it has no depth discrimination.

Pulsed Doppler instruments are designed to determine the distribution reflector velocities in the beam as a function of depth along the beam. The transmitter produces a pulse of energy, usually a short narrowband tone, which is reflected from the moving scatterers in the blood stream. The received echoes are processed in a variety of ways to deduce the Doppler shift as a function of depth along the beam. The frequency shift shown in Equation 2 is in the audio range, therefore the scattering positions must be measured with interrogating pulses at the appropriate sampling frequency, which is in the kilohertz range. Thus, the pulses must be sent into the tissue at a high pulse repetition rate to sample Doppler shifts (f_D) of the order of several kilohertz. The resulting signals can be processed in either the frequency domain by Fourier techniques, or in the time domain using correlation methods or less accurate methods such as zero crossing (12).

Frequency Domain

Doppler processing in the frequency domain consists of calculating the time-resolved Fourier transform at a fixed point in time along the received signal. The samples are obtained at the pulse repetition rate, and several methods are used to deduce the frequency distribution of the Doppler shift. Doppler frequencies are displayed in a variety of ways. They can be shown as a frequency versus time map or as a color distribution in a B-scan image.

Time Domain

Time domain methods of calculating the Doppler shift are becoming more popular. They use correlation methods to track the motion of scattered signals with time, and estimate their velocities (13,14). The advantages of these methods may be that they have different aliasing properties and can track faster motion.

DISPLAY

Display of the analyzed ultrasonic information is an important part of the medical imaging instrument. The echo signals are processed in a non-linear fashion to emphasize low-level signals while not discarding the high-level echoes from specular reflectors. The magnitude of the signal is displayed rather than the radio frequency amplitude. Directions of the beams in the tissue do not correspond to the rectangular arrangement of picture elements on the screen of the typical television monitor and therefore, interpolation from the arbitrary geometry of the ultrasonic samples in the tissue is used to match the geometry of the monitor's picture elements.

Scan Conversion

The geometry of the ultrasonic samples is converted from the geometry of the beams to that of the television monitor in a variety of ways, mostly using digital sampling and interpolation methods. The digital scan converter is now ubiquitous in medical imaging systems and provides TV resolution images with alpha numeric information such as patient I.D. and scan type, power levels, compression levels, etc., along with time and date of the examination. Modern instruments also provide color output to include Doppler information encoded into the B-scan information. Color is used to encode Doppler velocity and turbulence into the image of modern instruments. The information can be obtained from pulse Doppler and appropriate analyses of the signals.

Doppler velocity is often encoded in blue colors for velocities away from the ultrasonic probe and red colors for velocities toward the probe. Often, the user switches the colors to correspond to arterial flow or venous flow.

Turbulence is usually encoded into the Doppler colors using green; the more turbulent the measured velocity distribution, the greener the color. This method varies with manufacturer, however.

Trends

There are three especially active areas of research in ultrasonic imaging: elasticity imaging, three-dimensional imaging, and phase aberration correction.

Elasticity

Images of elasticity can be obtained by compressing the tissue while imaging with a scanner. Variations in the motion of the tissue give estimates of its stiffness much like palpation with the fingers, but with better resolution. Much effort is going into developing this method for clinical systems.

3-D

Three-dimensional imaging in ultrasound is being marketed by several companies. Methods include full three-dimensional arrays and mechanical motion or scanning of two-dimensional imaging planes. The sequential planes are arranged into a three-dimensional display in a computer.

Phase Correction

Phase aberrations caused by the inhomogeneities of speed within the tissue cause a limit to resolution available from the body. Several groups are trying to correct these aberrations by measuring them and adjusting the phase of the received signals across the image so that precise focusing is possible. The result should be much better focusing than currently available.

REFERENCES

1. Greenleaf JF. Tissue Characterization with Ultrasound. Vols I and II. Boca Raton: CRC Press Inc., 1986.
2. Sehgal CM, Lewallen DG, Robb RA, Greenleaf JF. Ultrasonic imaging of musculo-skeletal system. Int Union Physiol Sci 1991; 6:16–20.
3. Shung KK, Thieme GA. In: Ultrasonic Scattering in Biological Tissues. Boca Ratone: CRC Press Inc., 1993.
4. Haney MJ, O'Brien WD Jr. Temperature dependency of ultrasonic propagation proper-ties in biological materials. In: Greenleaf JF, ed. Tissue Characterization with Ultrasound. Vol. I. Boca Raton: CRC Press Inc., 1986:20.
5. Kino GS. Wave propagation with finite exciting sources. In: Acoustics Waves: Devices, Imaging, and Analog Signal Processing. Englewood Cliffs, NJ: Prentice-Hall Inc., 1987:154–317.
6. Wagner RF, Smith SW, Sandrik JM, Lopez H. Statistics of speckle in ultrasound B-scans. IEEE Trans Sonics Ultrason 1983; 30:156–173.
7. Ng GG, Worrell SS, Freiburger PD, Trahey GE. A comparative evaluation of several algorithms for phase aberration correction, IEEE Trans Ultrason, Ferroelec, Freq Contr 1994; 5(5); 41:631–642.
8. Smith WA. New opportunities in ultrasonic transducers emerging from innovations in piezoelectric materials. Proc SPIE 1992; 1733:3–26.
9. Tran HV, David T. A new selection criterion for piezoelectric transducer materials for optimal electro-acoustic power conservation. Proc SPIE 1992; 1733:78–90.
10. Goss SA, Frizzell LA, Dunn F. Ultrasonic absorption and attenuation in mammalian tissues. Ultrason Med Biol 1979; 5:181–186.
11. Fish PJ. Doppler methods. In: Hill CR, ed. Physical Principles of Medical Ultrasonics. Chichester, England: Ellis Horwood Limited, 1986:338–376.
12. Jones SA. Fundamental sources of error and spectral broadening to Doppler ultrasound signals. Clin Reviews Biomed Eng 1993; 21(5):399–483.
13. Tahey GE, Allison JW, Hubbard SM, Von Ramm OT. Measurement of local speckle pattern displacement to track blood flow in two dimensions. Proc IEEE Ultrason Symp 1987; 2:957–961.
14. Foster SG, Embree PM, O'Brien WD Jr. Flow velocity profile via time-domain correlation: Error analysis and computer simulation. IEEE Trans Ultrason, Ferroelec, Freq Contr 1990; 37:164–175.

2

Ultrasound Guidance for Central Venous Catheterization

Momen M. Wahidi
Interventional Pulmonology, Division of Pulmonary and
Critical Care Medicine, Department of Medicine, Duke University Medical Center, Durham,
North Carolina, U.S.A.

INTRODUCTION

The central venous catheter (CVC) is a valuable tool in the care of patients in both inpatient and outpatient settings. It facilitates the administration of fluids or medications in patients with difficult peripheral access and provides timely therapies to critically ill patients. Modified or tunneled catheters are now routinely used in ambulatory patients to offer chronic treatment such as hemodialysis or chemotherapy.

It is estimated that several million catheters are placed each year in the United States (1). CVCs are placed by physicians from a variety of specialties at various levels of training. Allied health professionals such as physician assistants and nurse practitioners have also joined the medical body capable of performing this procedure.

The classical method of CVC placement employs the landmark technique based on known anatomical relationship, which is between the vessel and surrounding tissue. The cut-down surgical technique, involving open surgical dissection to the level of the vein, is now a relic of the past and used only in extreme situations.

The complication rate for the landmark technique varies between 0.3% and 10% and depends on the selected insertion site, host factors, and operator's experience (1–3). Complications include: arterial puncture, subcutaneous hematoma, pneumothorax, hemothorax, mediastinal hematoma, nerve injury, arrhythmia, air embolus, and misplacement or failure of catheter placement.

Ultrasound (US) was introduced in 1978 as a guide for nonradiologists in the placement of CVC (4). Since then, numerous studies have been conducted addressing the merits and shortcomings of this US indication.

In this chapter, we will discuss the role of US in CVC placement in terms of technique, supporting data, current use, and future directions.

DEFINITIONS

Two types of US have been used in the guidance of CVC: Doppler and two-dimension US. Doppler US transforms the sound waves reflected from vessels into amplified audio signals. Arteries are recognized by their high-pitched pulsatile signal, while veins produce a lower-pitched signal that varies with respiration.

A variety of Doppler US devices have been devised including the fingertip-pulsed Doppler, probe-in-the-needle (SMART Needle, Peripheral System Group, Mountain View, California, U.S.A.), and the pencil-shaped probe (5–8).

Two-dimension US converts the sound waves reflected from tissue into a gray scale image, where vessels appear as tubular structures filled with hypoechoic "dark" blood. Arteries appear pulsatile and are noncompressible by applied pressure. Conversely, veins are non-pulsatile, easily compressible, and distensible with change in position (Trendelenburg) or maneuvers (Valsalva).

Guidance can be separated into sequential or real time. In the former, the vessel is localized by the US probe and a skin mark is placed on the optimal entry site. The probe is then removed and vein puncture proceeds without any further US aid.

Real-time guidance involves the use of US during the procedure where the probe is kept over the imaged vessel, and the puncturing needle is passed under direct visualization.

Most discussion in this chapter will center on real-time guidance with two-dimension US, since the sequential guidance technique and Doppler US have proved less beneficial.

ULTRASOUND AS AN IMAGING MODALITY FOR VESSELS

The advent of portable light-weight machines has made US a suitable modality for the guidance of CVC placement. The simplicity of US technology and the relative ease of learning how to decipher its images transported it from the realm of radiologists into the hands of medical practitioners.

The following benefits are attributed to US as a guiding tool in venous access. Whether or not the information gained from US translates into improvement in patient outcome will be discussed in a later section.

Precise Localization of the Vein and Artery

Visualization of the target vein allows its cannulation with a minimal number of needle passes and avoids inadvertent puncture of the adjacent artery (Figs. 1 and 2).

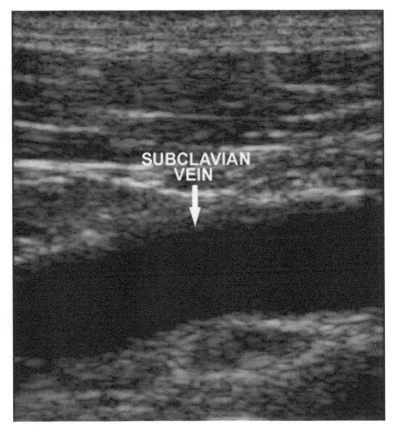

Figure 1
Sagittal and transverse two-dimension ultrasound view of the subclavian vein.

In studies of US applied to the necks of healthy volunteers, the internal jugular vein (IJV) was found to greatly vary in location based on the head position and neck rotation (9,10).

US localization of the vein achieves its highest benefits in patients with conditions that may cause difficulties in central venous access, such as morbid obesity, severe edema, inability to tolerate supine position, uncorrected coagulopathy, multiple previous catheterizations, and history of prior failed CVC insertion. Hatfield and Bodenham (11) used US in 33 patients with difficult or failed CVC placement and were able to locate an optimal site for catheterization in all the patients. Placement of central venous lines was then carried out in 22 of 31 of patients using real-time guidance and 9 of 31 using sequential guidance.

Detection of Anatomic Variation

A successful landmark technique relies on the expected location of the vein relative to the artery. Anatomic variations are uncommon but, when present, can significantly complicate the cannulation of central veins.

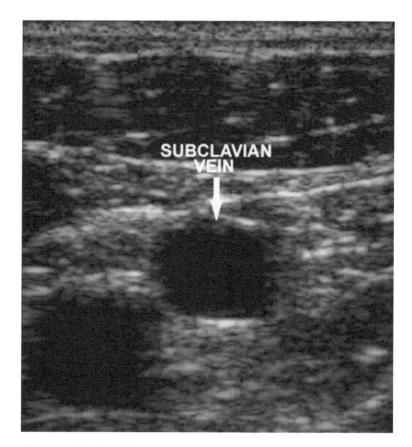

Figure 1 (*Continued*)
Transverse view.

Using two-dimension US, Denys and Uretsky (12) assessed the locations of the IJV and carotid artery (CA) in 200 patients undergoing placement of CVC. The IJV assumed the normal anatomical position, lateral and anterior to the CA, in 92% of patients, was >1 cm lateral to the CA in 1%, and medial to the CA in 2%. An interesting finding in this study was the discovery of unusually small IJV in 3% of patients, with no distensibility during the Valsalva maneuver.

Detection of Venous Thrombosis

Clotted veins are responsible for the frustrating occurrence of failure to advance the wire in the vessel despite an initial flash of blood. Clots can be detected as an echogenic shadow on direct ultrasonic visualization that impedes compressibility of the vein. Cannulation of a clotted vein is thus avoided with the aid of US and the effort is directed at another central vein.

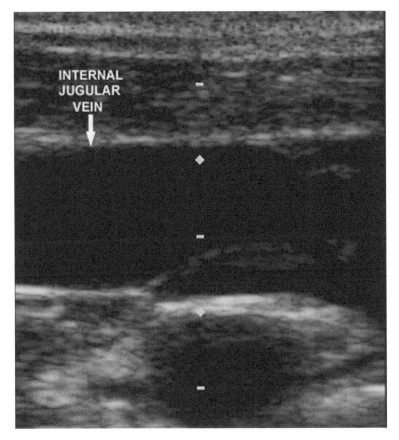

Figure 2
Sagittal and transverse two-dimension ultrasound view of the internal jugular vein.

TECHNICAL ASPECTS

The required instruments for US-guided placement of CVC include a US machine with a vascular probe, sterile plastic cover, sterile ultrasonic conductive medium, and a CVC kit.

A typical vascular US probe has a 7.5 MHz transducer, transversely-oriented tip, and a low depth (a range of 4–10 cm).

A kit containing a sterile cover, sterile US gel, and bands (to keep the sterile cover from sliding off the probe) is commercially available. When the specially designed sterile cover is not available, it can be substituted with sterile surgical gloves.

The patient is placed in the supine position and the site of insertion is selected: IJV, subclavian vein (SCV), or femoral vein (FV). The site is sterilized and draped in the usual fashion. The operator covers the US probe with a sterile plastic cover and applies sterile ultrasonic conductive gel to its tip. Other lubricating gels that are found in

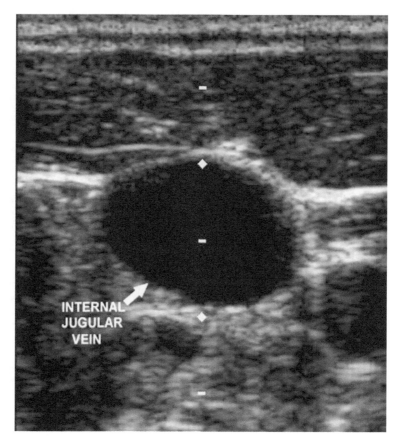

Figure 2 (*Continued*)
Transverse view.

examination rooms and medical wards are inferior in quality and produce poor US images.

Once the vein is located by displaying its characteristic qualities (compressibility and lack of pulsation), further confirmation is achieved by observing its distensibility; this is done by shifting the bed into a Trendelenburg position or asking the patient to perform a Valsalva maneuver. The US probe can be rotated over the vein to view it in either a transverse or a sagittal section. The sagittal view displays the needle within the vein more clearly. However, the transverse view is preferred for needle penetration as it shows the displacing effect of the advancing needle on the vein's surrounding tissue and its anterior wall. While locating the IJV and FV is fairly easy, finding the SCV is more technically challenging owing to the partial obstruction of the vein by the clavicle.

The US probe is kept over the located vein and a local anesthetic is applied to the subcutaneous tissue. The use of a smaller gauge "finding" needle is not required.

An 18-gauge needle is introduced at the cranial end of the probe and is advanced, under real guidance, through the anterior wall of the vein and into the lumen.

Some US probes are fitted with a ridge on their anterior surface where a disposable sterile needle guide can be mounted. In this case, the puncturing needle is advanced through the groove of the needle guide, allowing it to couple with the US probe and intersect in the center of the US image.

Occasionally, the vein can be seen collapsing under the pressure of the approaching needle; this causes the needle to pass through and beyond the vein with no return of blood. This explains the phenomenon of observing the "flash" of blood while the needle is seemingly being pulled away from the intended vein.

After the vein is punctured successfully, the US probe is removed and the procedure proceeds with the standard Seldinger technique.

US can be used to confirm the placement of the catheter within the lumen of the vessel. The catheter appears as a small tubular "white" shadow that is best appreciated in the sagittal US view (Fig. 3). Visualization of the catheter can be technically difficult, especially catheters with small diameters.

Care should be taken not to apply an excessive amount of conductive gel to the operative field; too much gel on the operator's hands renders the wire slippery and difficult to handle.

Although one operator can perform this procedure by steadying the US probe with one hand and controlling the needle with the other, the presence of two operators is ideal.

Newer US machines have the ability to register a patient's information, save ultrasonic images, and print selected images. Images of the scanned vein should be placed in the chart along with the operative report if possible.

EVIDENCE SUPPORTING THE USE OF ULTRASOUND IN CENTRAL VENOUS ACCESS

Numerous randomized clinical trials have been conducted to examine the role of US in central venous access and have reached varying conclusions (5,7,8,13–24). The patient populations were heterogeneous across the studies and the operators were, by necessity, not blinded to the intervention.

There is a general consensus that sequential US guidance is not superior to the landmark technique. This is mostly based on a large randomized trial by Mansfield et al. (1) where 821 patients in need of SCV catheterization were randomized to either sequential US guidance or standard insertion techniques. US guidance did not reduce the failure rate for SCV catheterization or incidence of complications.

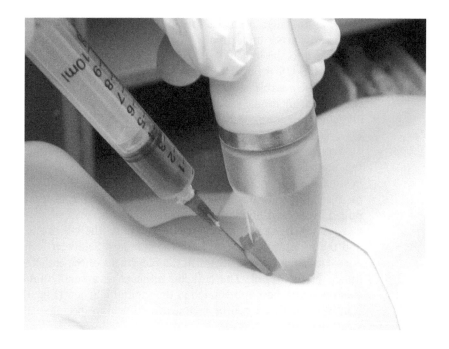

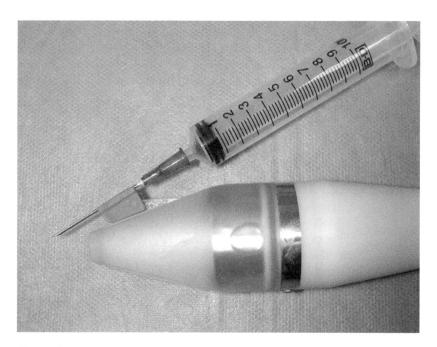

Figure 3
Set up for vein cannulation using an ultrasound probe equipped with needle
guide.

Two systematic reviews and meta-analyses have been carried out after summarizing the results of randomized clinical trials of real-time US guidance.

The first meta-analysis was conducted in 1996 by Randolph et al. (25). It identified eight clinical trials that fit predefined inclusion criteria. The trials addressed either Doppler or two-dimension US and assessed guidance for CVC placement in the IJV, SCV, or both. The results were in favor of real-time US guidance over the landmark technique: fewer CVC placement failures [relative risk (RR) 0.32; confidence interval (CI) 0.18–0.55], reduced number of catheter placement attempts (RR 0.60; CI 0.45–0.79), and fewer complications (RR 0.22; CI 0.10–0.45).

This meta-analysis has been criticized for pooling data from both Doppler and two-dimension US studies. Therefore, a second meta-analysis was conducted in the United Kingdom by Hind et al. (26). Eighteen studies were included with a total of 1646 patients. Data from Doppler and two-dimension US were analyzed separately.

Two-dimension US guidance was once again shown to reduce the number of catheter placement attempts and complications. The data were more compelling for the IJV site because only sparse data from small studies existed for SCV and FV sites. Similarly, Doppler US guidance improved the rate of successful CVC placement in the IJV site; however, it was inferior to the landmark technique in successful SCV catheter placement and proved to be more time consuming. No studies were found regarding Doppler US guidance for the FV site.

With respect to time to successful placement of CVC, the first meta-analysis found heterogeneous and inconclusive data, while the second demonstrated a time savings of 12 seconds with US guidance in the IJV site, a statistically significant difference of doubtful clinical benefit.

Operator experience is another worthy point of discussion. Benefits of US guidance were found for both experienced and inexperienced operators. In the three studies that focused on inexperienced operators, the benefits appeared more pronounced in this group of operators than their skilled counterparts; however, no scientific comparison has been undertaken to prove this observation (5,7,16).

The disparity in the benefits accrued from the use of sequential guidance versus real-time guidance is intriguing. Unlike stagnant organs like the pleural or peritoneal space where sequential US guidance prior to cavity puncture is beneficial, vessels are dynamic structures with constant change in lumen size and position based on temperature, blood pressure, volume status, respiratory variation, neck position, and skin tension (Fig. 4). This may explain the failure of sequential guidance and the need for moment-to-moment knowledge of the direction and position of the puncturing needle.

Cost is a significant concern with the routine use of US guidance in CVC placement. The health system will incur costs from purchase and maintenance of the US machine, as well as training of physicians and nurses. The cost might be offset by savings from reduction of complications and elimination of cost related to handling their sequelae

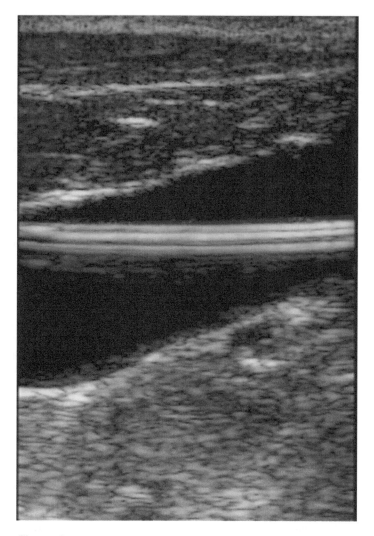

Figure 4
Sagittal and transverse two-dimension ultrasound view of catheter with the vein lumen.

such as extended hospital stays, operating room time, physician time, and expensive treatments.

A cost-effective economic evaluation of two-dimension real-time US guidance in central venous access, based on a spreadsheet decision-analytic model, was recently published (27). This report suggested a saving of $3249 for every 1000 procedures, assuming a sufficient use of the US machine of at least 15 times per week. More research is needed on the characteristics of the patients' population that would benefit the most from such an intervention, as well as its impact on mortality and quality of life.

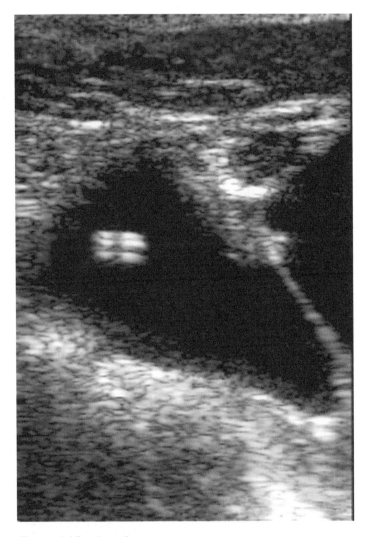

Figure 4 (*Continued*)
Transverse view.

CURRENT USE AND FUTURE DIRECTIONS

US enthusiasts have touted it as the "stethoscope of the millennium" and demanded its availability in every exam room.

It is not currently known how widespread the use of US in venous access guidance is in the United States. Information from the United Kingdom exists in the form of a survey of 176 critical care units: only 21.6% of them used US guidance with 11.1% using it routinely for every central line placement, 41.7% following failure of landmark technique, and 69.4% for an anticipated difficult vein cannulation (28). Units that did not use US guidance cited lack of equipment as the main reason (53%) followed by disbelief in its value (38.9%).

US guidance is endorsed by the Agency for Healthcare Research and Quality (AHRQ), a government agency in the United States that is charged with improving the quality of healthcare and patient safety (http://www.ahrq.gov/clinic/ptsafety/chap21.htm).

Similarly, a comparable agency in the United Kingdom, the National Institute for Clinical Excellence (NICE), has recommended the use of two-dimension US guidance as the preferred method for CVC placement in the IJV and advocated that all physicians involved in CVC placement get training in US and achieve competence (44). The NICE guidelines did not urge the use of US guidance in the SCV site and discouraged the use of Doppler US. These recommendations were met with skepticism and were widely debated in British medical journals (29–31).

Some have raised concerns about "de-skilling;" i.e., losing skills in the classical landmark technique of CVC placement by over-reliance on US guidance. However, the counter argument is that US guidance enhances the physician's knowledge of anatomical relationships between vessels and adjacent tissue, and boosts technical skills.

US guidance is now supported by reliable peer-reviewed data and it is only a matter of time until physicians believe in its credibility and add it to their armamentarium. What remains unforeseen is whether US guidance will be used routinely for every CVC placement or reserved for back up after failed attempts or for patients with anticipated difficult venous access.

OTHER USES OF ULTRASOUND IN VENOUS ACCESS

Peripherally inserted central catheters (PICC) have become a suitable, less-invasive alternative to CVC and have steadily gained popularity. An interventional radiology group reported the use of US as an adjunct to the placement of 355 PICCs in 262 patients (32). The overall success rate was 99% with an average of 1.2 punctures and occurrence of only two minor complications. This favorable experience was duplicated by intravenous nurse specialists in a study where US guidance led to a 42% decrease in the number of needle punctures necessary to cannulate the veins (33).

Another application of US is obtaining peripheral venous access in patients with "difficult" forearm veins (not appreciated by tactile palpation or direct vision) (34). Whiteley et al. (35) used Doppler US to study the audio signals of forearm veins in 12 "difficult" patients. The investigators classified the peripheral veins into "poor" or "good" and then verified this Doppler classification by measurement of the vein diameter with two-dimension US. The "good" veins had a mean diameter of 3.2 mm and were all amenable to percutaneous cannulation.

In addition to veins, radial arteries have been the subject of two small series in which Doppler US guidance facilitated arterial catheterization in hypotensive patients or those with impalpable peripheral arteries (36,37). A more recent study randomized patients undergoing radial artery catheterization to either two-dimension US guidance or palpation technique and had a higher cannulation rate on the first attempt in the US arm (62% vs. 34%) (38).

Finally, an innovative use of US as a diagnostic tool in the intensive care unit was suggested by Maury et al. (39). In this scenario, placement of CVC is performed using the landmark technique and US is used after placement to detect any resultant pneumothorax or catheter misplacement. US examination for this purpose took an average of 6.5 ± 3.5 minutes (as opposed to 80.3 ± 66.7 minutes for portable chest radiograph) and accurately identified the one case of pneumothorax and all but one case of misplacements. The results of this study are encouraging and have convenience, time and cost saving implications;e however, this US application requires advanced knowledge in ultrasonography to enable the operators to recognize the signs of pneumothorax in the pleural space and the undesirable distal location of the catheter tip in the heart chambers.

CREDENTIALING AND TRAINING

US is not currently a required element in nonradiology residency or fellowship training programs. Some trainees acquire basic US skills if US guidance for CVC placement is an adopted method at their institutions and is performed regularly on the medical wards or the intensive care units. Courses in US for nonradiologists are being offered in few academic medical centers or at national medial conferences. Educational software programs that cover various aspects of US are commercially available (40).

It has been shown that nonradiologist medical professionals can learn US and execute it accurately in focused examinations (41,42).

The objective of learning US for non-radiologists should focus on a basic understanding of US physics and machinery and procedure-specific targeted image interpretation. Complete diagnostic US evaluations are reserved for radiologists and are performed in dedicated suites with more sophisticated machines.

The ideal number of US-guided CVC placements to declare competency has not been studied. Judging from guidelines on other invasive procedures and given the relative simplicity of this technology, 10 procedures may be an adequate number to gain competency (43).

SUMMARY

Central venous access is an essential part of the care of patients in modern medicine. The landmark technique is a time-honored method that is highly successful when it is performed by an experienced operator on an average patient. Nevertheless, the rate of complications remains high, with minor complications causing significant patient discomfort and serious ones leading to considerable morbidity.

US guidance has emerged as an adjunct tool that can achieve successful placement of CVCs with fewer attempts and fewer complications. This methodology is now supported by a large body of evidence and will likely gain more acceptance among physicians as they acquire the necessary skills and realize its potential. Further research is necessary to weigh the effect of this technology on a patient's quality of life and mortality and to discover the circumstances where the benefit from its use is maximal.

REFERENCES

1. Mansfield PF, Hohn DC, Fornage BD, Gregurich MA, Ota DM. Complications and failures of subclavian-vein catheterization. N Engl J Med 1994; 331(26):1735–1738.
2. Bernard RW, Stahl WM. Subclavian vein catheterizations: a prospective study. I. Noninfectious complications. Ann Surg 1971; 173(2):184–190.
3. Sznajder JI, Zveibil FR, Bitterman H, Weiner P, Bursztein S. Central vein catheterization. Failure and complication rates by three percutaneous approaches. Arch Intern Med 1986; 146(2):259–261.
4. Ullman JI, Stoelting RK. Internal jugular vein location with the ultrasound Doppler blood flow detector. Anesth Analg 1978; 57(1):118.
5. Branger B, Zabadani B, Vecina F, Juan JM, Dauzat M. Continuous guidance for venous punctures using a new pulsed Doppler probe: efficiency, safety. Nephrologie 1994; 15(2):137–140.
6. Legler D, Nugent M. Doppler localization of the internal jugular vein facilitates central venous cannulation. Anesthesiology 1984; 60(5):481–482.
7. Gilbert TB, Seneff MG, Becker RB. Facilitation of internal jugular venous cannulation using an audio-guided Doppler ultrasound vascular access device: results from a prospective, dual-center, randomized, crossover clinical study. Crit Care Med 1995; 23(1):60–65.
8. Vucevic M, Tehan B, Gamlin F, Berridge JC, Boylan M. The SMART needle. A new Doppler ultrasound-guided vascular access needle. Anaesthesia 1994; 49(10):889–891.
9. Sulek CA, Gravenstein N, Blackshear RH, Weiss L. Head rotation during internal jugular vein cannulation and the risk of carotid artery puncture. Anesth Analg 1996; 82(1):125–128.
10. Armstrong PJ, Sutherland R, Scott DH. The effect of position and different manoeuvres on internal jugular vein diameter size. Acta Anaesthesiol Scand 1994; 38(3):229–231.
11. Hatfield A, Bodenham A. Portable ultrasound for difficult central venous access. Br J Anaesth 1999; 82(6):822–826.
12. Denys BG, Uretsky BF. Anatomical variations of internal jugular vein location: impact on central venous access. Crit Care Med 1991; 19(12):1516–1519.
13. Mallory DL, McGee WT, Shawker TH, Brenner M, Bailey KR, Evans RG, Parker MM, Farmer JC, Parillo JE. Ultrasound guidance improves the success rate of internal jugular vein cannulation. A prospective, randomized trial. Chest 1990; 98(1):157–160.
14. Troianos CA, Jobes DR, Ellison N. Ultrasound-guided cannulation of the internal jugular vein. A prospective, randomized study. Anesth Analg 1991; 72(6):823–826.
15. Gratz I, Afshar M, Kidwell P, Weiman DS, Shariff HM. Doppler-guided cannulation of the internal jugular vein: a prospective, randomized trial. J Clin Monit 1994; 10(3):185–188.
16. Gualtieri E, Deppe SA, Sipperly ME, Thompson DR. Subclavian venous catheterization: greater success rate for less experienced operators using ultrasound guidance. Crit Care Med 1995; 23(4):692–697.
17. Scherhag A, Klein A, Jantzen JP. Cannulation of the internal jugular vein using 2 ultrasonic technics. A comparative controlled study. Anaesthesist 1989; 38(11):633–638.
18. Bold RJ, Winchester DJ, Madary AR, Gregurich MA, Mansfield PF. Prospective, randomized trial of Doppler-assisted subclavian vein catheterization. Arch Surg 1998; 133(10):1089–1093.
19. Hilty WM, Hudson PA, Levitt MA, Hall JB. Real-time ultrasound-guided femoral vein catheterization during cardiopulmonary resuscitation. Ann Emerg Med 1997; 29(3):331–336.

20. Lefrant JY, Cuvillon P, Benezet JF, Dauzat M, Peray P, Saissi G, de La Coussaye JE, Eledjam JJ. Pulsed Doppler ultrasonography guidance for catheterization of the subclavian vein: a randomized study. Anesthesiology 1998; 88(5):1195–1201.

21. Nadig C, Leidig M, Schmiedeke T, Hoffken B. The use of ultrasound for the placement of dialysis catheters. Nephrol Dial Transplant 1998; 13(4):978–981.

22. Slama M, Novara A, Safavian A, Ossart M, Safar M, Fagon JY. Improvement of internal jugular vein cannulation using an ultrasound-guided technique. Intensive Care Med 1997; 23(8):916–919.

23. Sulek CA, Blas ML, Lobato EB. A randomized study of left versus right internal jugular vein cannulation in adults. J Clin Anesth 2000; 12(2):142–145.

24. Teichgraber UK, Benter T, Gebel M, Manns MP. A sonographically guided technique for central venous access. Am J Roentgenol 1997; 169(3):731–733.

25. Randolph AG, Cook DJ, Gonzales CA, Pribble CG. Ultrasound guidance for placement of central venous catheters: a meta-analysis of the literature. Crit Care Med 1996; 24(12):2053–2058.

26. Hind D, Calvert N, McWilliams R, Davidson A, Paisley S, Beverley C, Thomas S. Ultrasonic locating devices for central venous cannulation: meta-analysis. Br Med J 2003; 327(7411):361.

27. Calvert N, Hind D, McWilliams RG, Thomas SM, Beverley C, Davidson A. The effectiveness and cost-effectiveness of ultrasound locating devices for central venous access: a systematic review and economic evaluation. Health Technol Assess 2003; 7(12):1–84.

28. Jefferson P, Ogbue MN, Hamilton KE, Ball DR. A survey of the use of portable ultrasound for central vein cannulation on critical care units in the UK. Anaesthesia 2002; 57(4):365–368.

29. Chalmers N. Ultrasound guided central venous access. NICE has taken sledgehammer to crack nut. Br Med J 2003; 326(7391):712.

30. Bodenham AR. Ultrasound guided central venous access. Ultrasound localisation is likely to become standard practice. Br Med J 2003; 326(7391):712.

31. Muhm M. Ultrasound guided central venous access. Br Med J 2002; 325(7377):1373–1374.

32. Sofocleous CT, Schur I, Cooper SG, Quintas JC, Brody L, Shelin R. Sonographically guided placement of peripherally inserted central venous catheters: review of 355 procedures. Am J Roentgenol 1998; 170(6):1613–1616.

33. LaRue GD. Efficacy of ultrasonography in peripheral venous cannulation. J Intraven Nurs 2000; 23(1):29–34.

34. Mbamalu D, Banerjee A. Methods of obtaining peripheral venous access in difficult situations. Postgrad Med J 1999; 75(886):459–462.

35. Whiteley MS, Chang BY, Marsh HP, Williams AR, Manton HC, Horrocks M. Use of hand-held Doppler to identify 'difficult' forearm veins for cannulation. Ann R Coll Surg Engl 1995; 77(3):224–226.

36. Maher JJ, Dougherty JM. Radial artery cannulation guided by Doppler ultrasound. Am J Emerg Med 1989; 7(3):260–262.

37. Nagabhushan S, Colella JJ Jr, Wagner R. Use of Doppler ultrasound in performing percutaneous cannulation of the radial artery. Crit Care Med 1976; 4(6):327.

38. Levin PD, Sheinin O, Gozal Y. Use of ultrasound guidance in the insertion of radial artery catheters. Crit Care Med 2003; 31(2):481–484.

39. Maury E, Guglielminotti J, Alzieu M, Guidet B, Offenstadt G. Ultrasonic examination: an alternative to chest radiography after central venous catheter insertion? Am J Respir Crit Care Med 2001; 164(3):403–405.

40. Valley VT, Cardenas E, Spangler HM, Folstad S. Review of ultrasound educational CD-ROM software. Ann Emerg Med 1997; 29(3):375–379.

41. Buzzas GR, Kern SJ, Smith RS, Harrison PB, Helmer SD, Reed JA. A comparison of sonographic examinations for trauma performed by surgeons and radiologists. J Trauma 1998; 44(4):604–606.

42. Smith RS, Kern SJ, Fry WR, Helmer SD. Institutional learning curve of surgeon-performed trauma ultrasound. Arch Surg 1998; 133(5):530–535.

43. Ernst A, Silvestri GA, Johnstone D. Interventional pulmonary procedures: guidelines from the American College of Chest Physicians. Chest 2003; 123(5):1693–1717.

44. (http://www.nice.org.uk/pdf/ultrasound_49_GUIDANCE.pdf).

3

Ultrasound-Guided Thoracentesis

David Feller-Kopman
*Medical Procedure Service, Interventional Pulmonology, Beth Israel Deaconess Medical Center, Boston, Massachusetts, U.S.A.
and Harvard Medical School, Boston, Massachusetts, U.S.A.*

INTRODUCTION

Approximately 1.5 million people are found to have pleural effusions in the United States each year (1). Despite recent advances in ultrasound (US) technology, ultrasonography continues to be an underutilized modality in the evaluation of these patients, primarily limited to the reflection of US waves by bone and air. The acoustic window, therefore, is limited to the intercostal space. Fortunately, the presence of pleural fluid can be easily visualized and provides excellent contrast for pleura-based lesions on both the parietal and the visceral pleura. The advantages of US over standard chest radiography and computed tomography (CT) include the absence of radiation, portability, real-time imaging, and the ability to perform dynamic evaluations. US has also been found to be more sensitive than chest X-ray for the detection of pleural fluid (2) and, although slightly less sensitive than CT scanning, is easier to perform and can better distinguish pleural thickening from pleural effusion. Although there is a learning curve associated with the use of US, it is relatively short (3). Additionally, we routinely use ultrasonography as a teaching tool to reinforce the physical examination of residents and medical students (4).

TECHNICAL ASPECTS

Most authors recommend using a convex array 3.5 to 7.5 MHz probe when examining the thorax. The higher 5 to 7.5 MHz frequencies provide excellent resolution for chest wall and vascular structures (e.g., internal jugular vein), whereas the lower 3.5 to 5 MHz frequencies are ideal for visualizing deeper structures such as the pleural space (5). By convention, the groove on the transducer is directed cephalad, and the probe is moved along the superior–inferior axis as well as transversely across

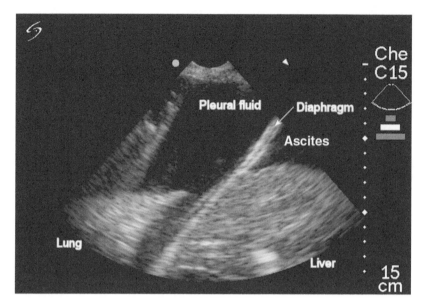

Figure 1
Overview of the pleural space. The hyperechoic, air-filled lung can be seen floating in anechoic pleural fluid. This patient has a large effusion causing flattening of the diaphragm. The echogenicity of the liver serves as a reference for echogenicity of other structures. Ascites can also be seen.

the chest, within the intercostal space. The skin and subcutaneous tissues are seen as multiple layers of soft-tissue echogenicity, and the parietal and visceral pleura are seen as two hyperechoic lines, typically <2 mm thick (6). The pleural space is visualized as a hypoechoic band approximately 0.3 mm in thickness, and therefore the exact identification of the pleura and pleural space, in the absence of pleural fluid, can sometimes be difficult (5,7). Air-filled lung is visualized as patterns of bright echoes caused by a reverberation artifact; as air enters the lung during inspiration, these echoes become brighter (more hyperechoic). Movement of the underlying lung with respiration produces a "sliding" or "gliding" sign, and this dynamic movement is utilized to help identify the visceral pleura and lung parenchyma. Diaphragmatic movement can also be visualized in real time, and is a key reference point when starting to perform US examination of the pleural space. The liver is used as an echo reference for the definition of hypo-, iso-, and hyperechoic reflections (Fig. 1). Pleural fluid is generally hypoechoic, and easily contrasts with the hyperechoic, air-filled lung. The ability of US to dynamically image the chest has proved beneficial in differentiating subpulmonic effusions from an elevated hemidiaphragm, and US is also nearly as sensitive as CT scanning in distinguishing atelectasis from effusion when the chest X-ray reveals opacification of the hemithorax (8).

ULTRASONOGRAPHIC FEATURES OF EFFUSIONS

Several studies have found that US can be helpful in identifying exudative effusions. Though an early study found that complex or septated fluid identified exudates in 74% of cases (9), more recent data suggest that effusions that are complex (either septated or nonseptated) or homogenously echoic are always exudates (10). Conversely, though transudates are almost always anechoic, anechoic fluid can be either transudative or exudative. Pleural thickening, in association with a parenchymal abnormality, also correlates with exudative fluid, and homogenously echogenic effusions are typically seen with hemorrhage or empyema (10). Sonographic septation has been found to predict the need for pleural interventions such as intrapleural fibrinolysis or surgical debridement, as well as be associated with an increased duration of chest tube drainage and hospital stay (Fig. 2) (11). Another sonographic finding, the echogenic swirling pattern, describes multiple echogenic particles within a pleural effusion that move with respiratory or cardiac motion (12). Although this can be seen in patients with or without malignancy, in patients with underlying malignancy, this pattern is associated with the presence of malignant pleural effusion.

The volume of fluid in the pleural space can also be sonographically estimated, and when examining patients who are in the supine position, the volume of fluid seen on US correlates better with actual fluid volume than the amount of fluid estimated from a lateral decubitus chest X-ray (13). An important point in using this method of evaluating pleural fluid volume is that the transducer must be perpendicular to the chest, as an oblique angle will over- or underestimate the volume. Another caveat of this method is the fact that a larger thoracic volume will distribute a given amount of fluid over a larger area, and therefore reduce the estimated volume seen sonographically.

As pleural thickening can be anechoic, the sole presence of an echo-free space does not guarantee the presence of pleural fluid. Dynamic changes, including the change of shape with respiratory movement, or the presence of movable echo densities, are therefore considered the sine qua non of pleural fluid (14). Some authors advocate the use of the fluid "color signal," the change in color seen during respiratory or cardiac motion, to identify small or loculated effusions (15,16).

US has also been evaluated in patients with "white out" of a hemithorax. Using CT as the gold standard, US has been found to have a 95% sensitivity for detecting pleural lesions in this group of patients (8). As one would expect, the ability of US to detect parenchymal or mediastinal pathology is significantly limited when compared to CT. Clear benefits of US, when compared to CT scanning, include its portability, low cost, lack of radiation exposure, and ability to perform real-time procedural guidance.

A

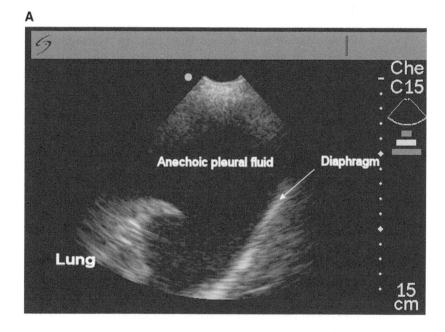

B

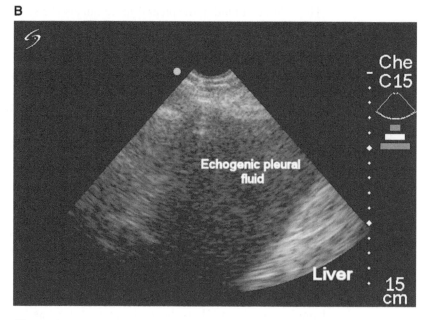

Figure 2

Variations in the ultrasonographic appearance of pleural fluid. (**A**) The hyper-echoic lung surrounded by anechoic fluid. This patient had a transudative effu-sion from congestive heart failure. (**B**) Homogenously echogenic pleural fluid. This patient had a hemothorax. (**C**) Loculations in the pleural space from empyema. (**D**) Enhancement of the visceral pleura secondary to prior pleural inflammation resulting in trapped lung.

C

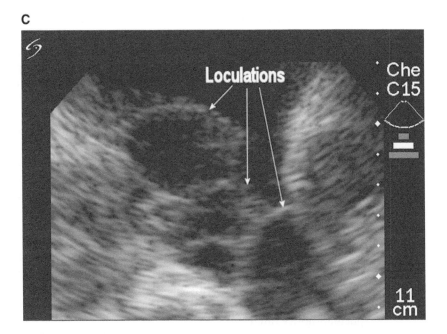

D

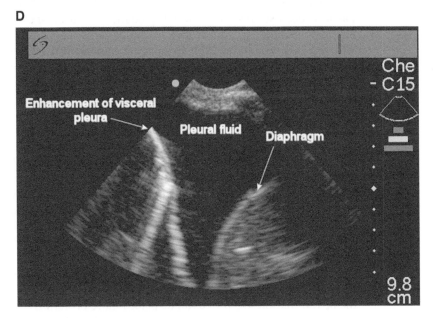

Figure 2   *(Continued)*

GUIDANCE FOR THORACENTESIS

Thoracentesis is typically thought to be a relatively safe procedure with few complications. The incidence of pneumothorax, however, has been reported to be as high as 20% to 39% (17). Procedural factors that have been shown to reduce the rate of pneumothorax include the performance by experienced personnel (18) and the use of US (17,19,20). Additionally, when the size of the effusion is less than one-half of the hemithorax, the probability of obtaining adequate fluid samples can be significantly improved when compared to relying on the lateral decubitus film alone (21).

Grogan et al. (17) found a significant reduction in the pneumothorax rate when US was utilized for identification of needle placement (0% vs. approximately 29%). Likewise, in a study by Raptopoulos et al. (20), the rate of pneumothorax complicating thoracentesis was 3% when ultrasound was utilized, as compared with 18% when the effusion was localized clinically. This held true whether the amount of pleural fluid was deemed small or large, whether the thoracenteses were diagnostic or therapeutic, and whether the tap was "dry" or "near dry." The occurrence of pneumothorax requiring tube thoracotomy was also significantly reduced with US guidance (2% vs. 7%). Interestingly, the "X marks the spot" technique, i.e., having a radiologist use US to mark the needle insertion site with the thoracentesis performed when the patient returned to the floor, was not associated with a reduction in the pneumothorax rate (20).

The utility of US after a failed clinically directed thoracentesis has also been studied, and the US guidance has been shown to obtain adequate samples in almost half of the patients who had a "dry tap" with the X-ray method (21). Even more impressively, two recent studies suggest that fluid can be successfully obtained in approximately 88% of patients after unsuccessful clinically guided thoracenteses (9,22). Perhaps even more importantly, in 58% of clinically attempted thoracenteses, the needle insertion site found to be below the diaphragm (22).

Critical care physicians can easily acquire the sonography skills required to guide thoracentesis in the intensive care unit (ICU), and do so without radiology support (3). In a prospective analysis of 232 US-guided thoracenteses in patients requiring mechanical ventilation, only three (1.3%) developed a pneumothorax (3). For patients in the ICU, we generally scan the lateral chest wall with the patient supine and the ipsilateral arm brought over the chest to the opposite side. As always, the groove on the transducer is directed cephalad. This position is easiest for the patient and the nurse, and moderate effusions can easily be seen. With smaller effusions, we slide the patient closer to the edge of the bed so that the US probe can be placed more posteriorly. It is uncommon for us to sit the patient upright—a task that often requires at least two assistants for patients requiring mechanical ventilation.

PNEUMOTHORAX

Although a pneumothorax is easily seen using conventional chest X-ray or chest CT, the portability of US, especially when used at the point of care, makes this technology especially useful for identifying a postprocedural pneumothorax. US characteristics of pneumothorax include the loss of the gliding lung sign as well as the loss of "comet tail" artifacts (23). The "comet tail" artifacts are due to echo reverberations of the air-filled lung, and appear as narrow hyperechoic, ray-like opacities extending from the pleural line to the edge of the ultrasound screen. The gliding lung typically is best seen anteriorly, over the midcaudal thorax where lung displacement during respiration is greatest. Because air will travel to the least dependent position, this examination should be performed with the patient supine. As adhesions or diaphragmatic paralysis may limit lung sliding, the main utility of US for assessment of pneumothorax relates to its ability to rule out a pneumothorax; that is, the presence of lung sliding rules out a pneumothorax although the absence of lung sliding does not mean a pneumothorax is present. Although US can rule out a pneumothorax, it cannot quantitate its size when present, and standard radiographs are required.

SUMMARY

Ultrasonography is an easily learned procedure that not only enhances the physical examination, but also has the distinct advantage of being a portable tool that can provide real-time evaluation of the pleural space. Its use has been associated with an improved yield and reduced complication rate for thoracentesis, and it is quickly becoming the standard of care for procedural guidance.

REFERENCES

1. Light RW. Pleural Diseases. 4th. Philadelphia: Lippincott Williams & Wilkins, 2001.
2. Gryminski J, Krakowka P, Lypacewicz G. The diagnosis of pleural effusion by ultrasonic and radiologic techniques. Chest 1976; 70(1):33–37.
3. Mayo PH, Goltz HR, Tafreshi M, Doelken P. Safety of ultrasound-guided thoracentesis in patients receiving mechanical ventilation. Chest 2004; 125(3):1059–1062.
4. Rozycki GS, Pennington SD, Feliciano DV. Surgeon-performed ultrasound in the critical care setting: its use as an extension of the physical examination to detect pleural effusion. J Trauma 2001; 50(4):636–642.
5. Beckh S, Bolcskei PL, Lessnau KD. Real-time chest ultrasonography: a comprehensive review for the pulmonologist. Chest 2002; 122(5):1759–1773.
6. Mathis G. Thoraxsonography—Part I: Chest wall and pleura. Ultrasound Med Biol 1997; 23(8):1131–1139.
7. Tsai TH, Yang PC. Ultrasound in the diagnosis and management of pleural disease. Curr Opin Pulm Med 2003; 9(4):282–290.
8. Yu CJ, Yang PC, Wu HD, Chang DB, Kuo SH, Luh KT. Ultrasound study in unilateral hemithorax opacification. Image comparison with computed tomography. Am Rev Respir Dis 1993; 147(2):430–434.
9. Hirsch JH, Rogers JV, Mack LA. Real-time sonography of pleural opacities. Am J Roentgenol 1981; 136(2):297–301.
10. Yang PC, Luh KT, Chang DB, Wu HD, Yu CJ, Kuo SH. Value of sonography in determining the nature of pleural effusion: analysis of 320 cases. Am J Roentgenol 1992; 159(1):29–33.
11. Chen KY, Liaw YS, Wang HC, Luh KT, Yang PC. Sonographic septation: a useful prognostic indicator of acute thoracic empyema. J Ultrasound Med 2000; 19(12):837–843.
12. Chian CF, Su WL, Soh LH, Yan HC, Perng WC, Wu CP. Echogenic swirling pattern as a predictor of malignant pleural effusions in patients with malignancies. Chest 2004; 126(1):129–134.
13. Eibenberger KL, Dock WI, Ammann ME, Dorffner R, Hormann MF, Grabenwoger F. Quantification of pleural effusions: sonography versus radiography. Radiology 1994; 191(3):681–684.
14. Marks WM, Filly RA, Callen PW. Real-time evaluation of pleural lesions: new observations regarding the probability of obtaining free fluid. Radiology 1982; 142(1):163–164.
15. Wu RG, Yang PC, Kuo SH, Luh KT. "Fluid color" sign: a useful indicator for discrimination between pleural thickening and pleural effusion. J Ultrasound Med 1995; 14(10):767–769.
16. Wu RG, Yuan A, Liaw YS, Chang DB, Yu CJ, Wu HD, Kuo SH, Luh KT, Yang PC. Image comparison of real-time gray-scale ultrasound and color Doppler ultrasound for use in diagnosis of minimal pleural effusion. Am J Respir Crit Care Med 1994; 150(2):510–514.
17. Grogan DR, Irwin RS, Channick R, Raptopoulos V, Curley FJ, Bartter T, Corwin RW. Complications associated with thoracentesis. A prospective, randomized study comparing three different methods. Arch Intern Med 1990; 150(4):873–877.
18. Bartter T, Mayo PD, Pratter MR, Santarelli RJ, Leeds WM, Akers SM. Lower risk and higher yield for thoracentesis when performed by experienced operators. Chest 1993; 103(6):1873–1876.
19. Jones PW, Moyers JP, Rogers JT, Rodriguez RM, Lee YC, Light RW. Ultrasound-guided thoracentesis: is it a safer method? Chest 2003; 123(2):418–423.

20. Raptopoulos V, Davis LM, Lee G, Umali C, Lew R, Irwin RS. Factors affecting the development of pneumothorax associated with thoracentesis. Am J Roentgenol 1991; 156(5):917–920.
21. Kohan JM, Poe RH, Israel RH, Kennedy JD, Benazzi RB, Kallay MC, Greenblatt DW. Value of chest ultrasonography versus decubitus roentgenography for thoracentesis. Am Rev Respir Dis 1986; 133(6):1124–1126.
22. Weingardt JP, Guico RR, Nemcek AA Jr, Li YP, Chiu ST. Ultrasound findings following failed, clinically directed thoracenteses. J Clin Ultrasound 1994; 22(7):419–426.
23. Targhetta R, Bourgeois JM, Chavagneux R, Coste E, Amy D, Balmes P, Pourcelot L. Ultrasonic signs of pneumothorax: preliminary work. J Clin Ultrasound 1993; 21(4):245–250.

4

Ultrasound-Guided Percutaneous Drainage

F. J. F. Herth
Department of Pneumology and Critical Care Medicine, Thoraxklinik, University of Heidelberg, Heidelberg, Germany

This chapter discusses real-time ultrasound ultrasound-guided percutaneous drainage for the practicing pulmonologist. Ultrasound (US) supplements chest radiography and chest computed tomography (CT) scanning. Major advantages include bedside availability, absence of radiation, and guided aspiration of fluid-filled areas and solid tumors (1). Additionally, pulmonary vessels and vascular supply of consolidations may be visualized without contrast. US may help to diagnose conditions such as pneumothorax, hemothorax, and pleural or pericardial effusion (2). The technique of therapeutic US is cost effective compared to CT scanning and magnetic resonance imaging (MRI), and may be learned relatively easily by the pulmonologist (3). Percutaneous catheter drainage of intrathoracic collections has developed as a natural extension of similar interventional radiology procedures in the abdomen (4,5). The advent of CT and sonography, which allow detection and characterization of pleural and parenchymal collections, combined with advances in drainage catheter design and interventional techniques, has made image-guided management of intrathoracic collections a safe and effective alternative to traditional surgical therapy (6). Though we routinely use image guidance for the placement of PleurX™ (Denver Biomedical, Inc., Golden, Colorado, U.S.A.) catheters in patients with malignant pleural effusions, this chapter specifically discusses issues related to percutaneous drainage of empyema, lung abscess, and pneumothorax.

MALIGNANT EFFUSIONS

Malignant disease accounts for nearly one-half of all exudative pleural effusions in patients undergoing thoracentesis (Fig. 1) (9). Approximately 75% of these malignant effusions are due to lung and breast carcinoma and lymphoma (10). The presence of malignant cells on cytologic examination of pleural fluid or presence of tumor implants on pleural biopsy is necessary for diagnosis. Whereas some effusions resolve with treatment

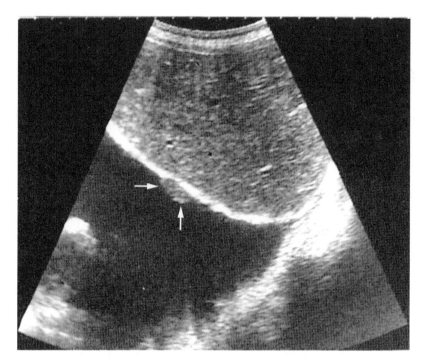

Figure 1
Metastasis (*arrows*) on the diaphragm and moderate pleural effusion.

of the underlying malignancy (e.g., small-cell carcinoma or lymphoma), the majority will require external drainage. Although therapeutic large-volume thoracentesis is appropriate in selected patients with a short life expectancy, 97% of patients need a repeat therapeutic thoracentesis at one month (11). The latter type of patients require drainage and obliteration of the pleural space, which can be accomplished with either thoracoscopy and pleurodesis or placement of a long-term drainage catheter (e.g., PleurX^{TM}). The catheter is placed using sterile technique under local lidocaine anesthesia. The entry site into the pleural space is marked by US and, using the modified Seldinger technique, a guidewire is inserted into the pleural space. The catheter is then tunneled subcutaneously, and passed over the guidewire into the effusion.

PARAPNEUMONIC EFFUSIONS/EMPYEMAS

Infected pleural fluid collections most often develop as a complication of pulmonary infection, chest trauma, or recent surgery, or as secondary infection of a pre-existing hydrothorax or hemothorax (12). A para-pneumonic pleural effusion develops in approximately 40% of patients with community-acquired pneumonia (13). Most of these collections resolve with appropriate antibiotic therapy directed toward the causative organism. Effusions that require drainage for definitive treatment are termed "complicated parapneumonic effusions." Some complicated parapneumonic effusions can be further described as an "empyema" (14,15). Anaerobic and mixed aerobic–anaerobic infections have become the most common cause of complicated parapneumonic effusions in the last two decades as a result of the widespread use of broad-spectrum antistaphylococcal and antistreptococcal antibiotics (13).

A variety of echo patterns may be present with empyema. In a study of 320 cases of pleural effusions, Yang et al. (4) found empyema as homogeneously echogenic. In most cases, septations and multiple moving and swirling reflections correlate with increased protein or cells. Thickened walls surround empyema. Using real-time US, the contiguous lung parenchyma usually is fixed to the inflamed areas. The US findings may be important for decision making about treatment and in reducing hospitalization (16,17). In a study by Ramnath et al. (16), patients with septations or loculations seen on US did not benefit from drainage procedures and required decortication. A CT scan helps to distinguish between abscess and empyema (Fig. 2A–C) (18,19). With lobulated empyema, the CT scan reveals the entire spatial extent. External drainage of infected pleural fluid collections has been the mainstay of treatment for centuries (18).

LUNG ABSCESS

Primary lung abscess usually results from aspiration of anaerobic oropharyngeal bacteria into gravity-dependent portions of the lung, most often in the posterior segments of the upper lobes and the superior segments of the lower lobes. It is seen most commonly in alcoholics and other persons with altered consciousness, patients with gastroesophageal dysmotility, and those with poor dental status (20,21). Most abscesses are discovered when fever and pulmonary symptoms lead to a chest radiograph that reveals a solid or cavitary lung mass (19,22).

Lobar pneumonia, segmental pneumonia affecting the pleura, and pleura-based consolidation are detectable on US. In general, the size of the pneumonia appears smaller on US than on radiographs (23). This is because the periphery of the pneumonia is more air-filled, which results in more artifacts, thus limiting complete visualization of the extent of consolidation.

In the early phase of consolidation, the lung appears diffusely echogenic, resembling the sonographic texture of the liver. The shape of the pneumonia is rarely well defined, often showing irregular or serrated outlines. Branching echogenic structures are often seen (87% of patients) within the pneumonia and represent air bronchograms. Multiple lenticular echoes, representing air inlets and measuring a few millimeters in diameter and extending to the pleural surface, are also frequently observed. These lenticular echoes vary with respiration (7,24,25).

Fluid bronchograms may also be observed sonographically in patients with pneumonia (16–92%) (3). These are identified as anechoic tubular structures, representing fluid-filled airways. The fluid broncho-gram is seen in bronchial obstruction, which can result from either impacted secretions or a proximal tumor (24,25). Although the fluid bronchogram may be seen in isolated pneumonia, the presence of this sign in the appropriate clinical context should raise the suspicion of postobstructive pneumonitis. Indeed, US may be able to help in distin-guishing the central obstructing tumor as a hypoechoic mass from the distal, more echogenic consolidation (25).

As the disease progresses, the echogenicity of the pneumonia increases and becomes more heterogeneous. With successful treatment, re-established ventilation within the consolidation gives rise to more air-inlet artifacts, and the area of pneumonia diminishes in size. Pneumonia resulting from pyogenic organisms can undergo necrosis leading to lung abscess formation. A lung abscess can be identified on US as a hypoechoic

A

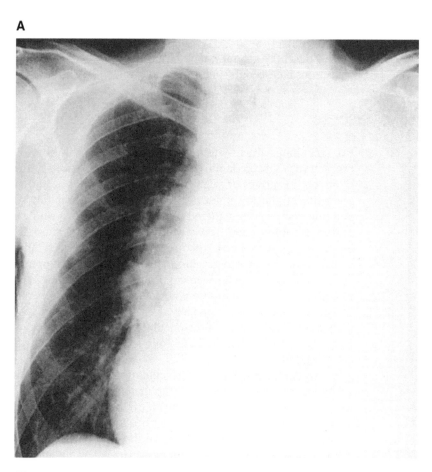

Figure 2
(**A**) *Chest X-ray.* Complete opacity of the left hemithorax. (**B**) *CT scan.* Homogeneous mass with prominent walls. (**C**) *US.* Inhomogeneous echogenic effusion. Puncture produced purulent fluid. *Abbreviations*: A, effusion; Ao, aorta; Cor, heart; CT, computed tomography; US, ultrasound.

B

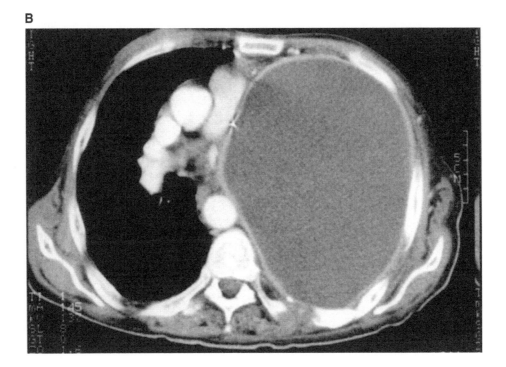

C

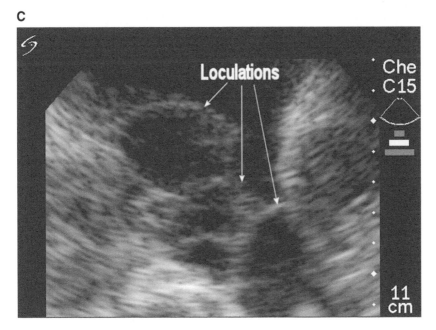

Figure 2 *(Continued)*

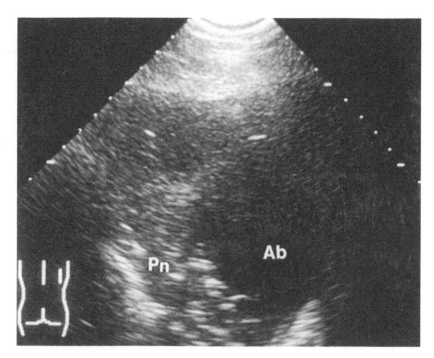

Figure 3
Lung abcess. *Abbreviations*: Ab, abscess; Pn, infiltrated lung.

lesion with a well defined or irregular wall (26,27). The center of the abscess is usually anechoic but may contain internal echoes and septations (5).

Until the early 1940s, surgical pneumonotomy and drainage were the accepted treatments for lung abscess (20). Subsequent advances in anesthesia and surgical techniques led to the advent of lung resection as the preferred therapy, until the availability of effective antibiotics rendered open drainage unnecessary in most patients (21). The current first-line therapy for lung abscess is antibiotic therapy directed at the likely causative organisms, usually anaerobes or mixed aerobic and anaerobic bacteria (28).

Conservative medical therapy proves effective in 80% to 90% of patients with lung abscess (29,30). Patients who display no radiographic evidence of improvement or who show signs of persistent sepsis or develop complications such as hemoptysis or bronchopleural fistula and empyema, require external drainage or resection for definitive treatment. External drainage is the preferred method of treatment for pleura-based abscesses, particularly in patients with a high risk of surgical mortality. Sonography-guided percutaneous drainage has been successfully used for the treatment of lung abscess (Fig. 3) (28). Placement of a relatively large-bore catheter (12-French or greater diameter) is key to establishing adequate external drainage and maintaining catheter patency. Once the catheter is positioned in the abscess cavity, fluid is aspirated manually, and the cavity is irrigated with saline. The drainage catheter is placed to suction at –20 cm of water to help evacuate pus and collapse the cavity. The catheter should be irrigated with sterile saline at least twice daily to maintain patency. When daily assessment by clinical parameters (temperature, WBC count) and chest radiographs indicates resolution of the abscess, the catheter may be removed. A repeat CT scan is obtained when there is lack of improvement, particularly if a complicating bronchopleural fistula and empyema are present (28–30).

Several investigators have reported their results of image-guided percutaneous drainage of lung abscess (19,20,28,31). In the largest series published to date, van Sonnenberg et al. (18) reported successful percutaneous lung abscess drainage in all 19 patients referred for this procedure, with surgery avoided in 16 patients (84%). Mean time to abscess resolution is approximately 10 to 15 days, although a marked improvement in sepsis indicators (fever, leukocytosis) is seen within 48 hours of drainage (18,30). Potential percutaneous abscess drainage complications are pneumothorax, bronchopleural fistula formation with empyema, and hemorrhage. Alternatives to the percutaneous approach are also bronchoscopically placed catheters via the nasal route (31,32).

PNEUMOTHORAX

Pneumothorax may be traumatic or spontaneous. Traumatic pneumothorax most often results from penetrating or blunt chest trauma, or as an iatrogenic complication of thoracentesis, central venous catheterization, or transbronchial/transthoracic needle lung biopsy. Spontaneous pneumothorax may be divided into a primary form, which has no identifiable cause and is often related to apical intrapleural bleb rupture, and a secondary form, which is associated with underlying parenchymal lung disease.

Patients with small, stable pneumothoraces are safely observed on bed rest with administration of supplemental oxygen. Indications for pneumothorax drainage include collections estimated to exceed 25% of the volume of one hemithorax, an enlarging pneumothorax indicating persistent air leak, or a pneumothorax of any size that causes dyspnea or severe chest pain (33). An additional indication for pneumothorax drainage is a transthoracic needle biopsy complicated by pneumothorax (34). Patients with recurrent pneumothorax or persistent bronchopleural fistula may require more than simple chest tube drainage, including tube thoracostomy with chemical pleurodesis, thoracoscopic talc poudrage, or even thoracotomy with bullectomy (34,35).

The reader is referred to Chapter 3 for a review of the ultrasonographic features of pneumothorax. Pneumothorax drainage using small-gauge catheters is easily performed under sonographic guidance. In most patients, an anterior approach through the second intercostal space in the mid-clavicular line is used to direct the catheter into the pleural apex. Once an intrapleural position is confirmed by aspirating air through the hollow trocar, the catheter/trocar combination is advanced an additional 1 cm to be certain the catheter tip is intrapleural. The catheter is then advanced and taped or sutured to the skin, and the pneumothorax is manually aspirated with a large syringe until resistance is encountered. The catheter is then attached via an adapter to an underwater seal device with suction or to a Heimlich valve. If the lung remains re-expanded, the catheter is removed (35–37). Patients with prolonged air leaks and incomplete re-expansion of the lung may require thoracoscopic or open procedures.

The success of image-guided drainage of postbiopsy pneumothorax using catheters from 5.5- to 16-French in outer diameter is 87% to 93% (34,38,39), with mean duration of pleural drainage being approximately three days. Pneumothorax drainage failure may be due to catheter kinking or occlusion by blood or fibrin (37), inadvertent withdrawal from the pleural space, or presence of a large air leak (34).

TECHNIQUE OF ULTRASOUND-GUIDED DRAINAGE

Fluoroscopy, sonography, CT, or any combination of these techniques can accurately guide drainage catheter placement (40). Image guidance is selected by: (i) availability and convenience of the various techniques, (ii) size and position of the collection, (iii) the patient's condition, and (iv) the physician's preference. Continuous monitoring of the course of the needle, guidewire, and catheter is a distinct advantage of fluoroscopy.

These procedures are best performed in an interventional suite, where immediate access to any necessary wires and catheters is available. Image-guided catheter placement has largely replaced surgical thoracostomy tube as the initial procedure of choice for management of effusions. Because most effusions are free flowing, they are easily accessed for catheter drainage by sonographic examination with placement of the drainage catheter in the dependent portion of the pleural space (41–43).

The puncture may be performed in a sitting position if the patient is unable to lie supine. The patient should be placed in a position that will prevent sudden movement of the chest. The area of the planned drainage placement is cleaned with disinfecting solution which may also be used as the transmitting medium instead of nonsterile sono-gel. Any solution may be used as long as it does not destroy the surface of the relatively expensive transducer (1,2,22). Several commercially available US probe covers with sterile gel are also available.

Successful pleural space drainage requires careful attention to technique and familiarity with drainage devices. In a patient with suspected pleural space infection, a diagnostic thoracentesis is performed initially under sonographic guidance. Once the puncture site has been sterilely prepared and anesthetized, an 18-gauge needle is placed through the chest wall into the thickest part of the collection (Figs. 4 and 5A,B). The needle should be superior to an underlying rib to avoid injury to the intercostal vessels and nerve. If pus is obtained, a drainage catheter is placed. Nonpurulent fluid

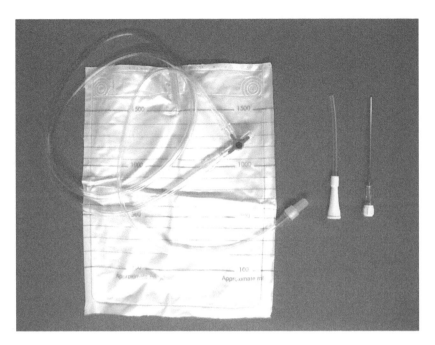

Figure 4
Pleura drainage set.

should be sent for immediate Gram's stain to identify microorganisms, and the presence of organism warrants catheter drainage.

Catheter insertion can be accomplished by placing a J-tipped guidewire through the needle, into the collection. The needle is then removed and sequential vascular dilators in increments of 2-French are placed over the wire until the drainage catheter diameter is reached. The drainage catheter is placed over the guidewire and into the dependent part of the collection. Tapered pigtail catheters are also available which can also be threaded over the guidewire. Collections with a large window of safety are easily drained by trocar placement of the drainage catheter in tandem with the diagnostic needle (Figs. 6A,B). Once the catheter has been placed to the appropriate depth, the inner sharp-tipped trocar is removed through the lumen of the stiffening inner cannula, and fluid is aspirated to confirm accurate catheter placement. The catheter is then advanced off the cannula into the collection (4,8,27). Fluid is then manually aspirated until mild resistance is encountered. A repeat sonogram scan through the area of interest can assess drainage adequacy (Fig. 7). If there are undrained locules, additional catheters can be placed. Catheters are then affixed to the skin and attached via an adapter to a suction device.

Catheters ranging from 8- to 30-French in outer diameter may be placed under imaging guidance. A single-lumen catheter should be used to prevent air entry into the pleural space, which would impair lung

A

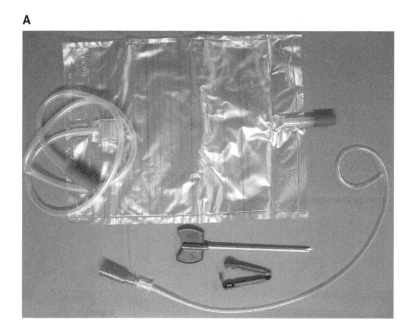

B

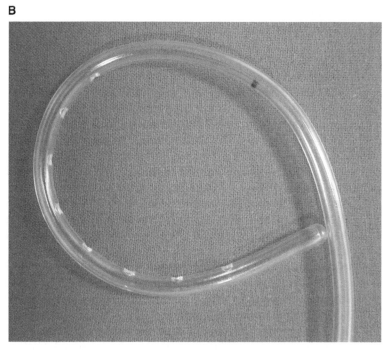

Figure 5
(**A**) Pleura drainage set (Trokar technique); (**B**) Tip of the pigtail catheter.

re-expansion and obliteration of the empyema cavity. For serous collections, a 10- or 12-French catheter provides adequate drainage; thick collections of purulent or bloody material may require catheters 24- to 28-French in diameter. Most empyema drainage tubes have large round or oval side holes to promote drainage of particulate matter. The catheter tip may be either pigtail shaped or gently curved to conform to the inner concavity of the pleural space. A potential advantage of the pigtail catheter is the reduced risk of injuring the underlying parenchyma.

A recent review found small-bore catheters (8–14-French) to be effective in treatment for parapneumonic effusion, empyema, malignant effusion, and pneumothorax (43). The smaller tubes are also much better tolerated than the large-bore intercostal chest drains that have traditionally been used by clinicians for the initial treatment of parapneumonic effusions. Image-guided placement of small-bore catheters has been successful in the treatment of empyema (44). Small-bore catheters are also associated with a lower complication rate compared with that of the large-bore chest drains (43).

The patient is visited daily to assess therapeutic response and catheter patency maintained by flushing the catheter with small amounts of sterile saline. Duration of catheter drainage following image-guided placement ranges from 1 to 45 days, with most requiring 5 to 10 days of treatment (23–27). The drainage catheter should be removed when drainage has diminished to less than 10 mL daily, the patient's fever and WBC count have diminished, and sonographic resolution of the pleural collection has occurred.

Several options exist if clinical and radiographic assessment determines that drainage is inadequate. Occasionally, the indwelling catheter requires repositioning to enhance drainage. Conversion to a catheter with a larger diameter may promote adequate drainage of thick pus or bloody material. Intrapleural administration of fibrinolytic medication may aid in septated collections or collections with multiple locules. Both streptokinase and urokinase have been used successfully to avoid open procedures in patients in whom simple closed thoracostomy catheter drainage has failed. Several investigators have reported the use of 80,000 to 100,000 IU of urokinase mixed in 100 mL of sterile water or saline administered through the indwelling catheter and left in the pleural space for 2 to 12 hours before replacing the catheter to suction (45–47). The success rate in these small series of selected patients was 77%. Despite these maneuvers, the decision to proceed to thoracoscopy or open surgical drainage should be made when more conservative measures fail and there is clinical evidence of persistent pleural infection and sepsis.

TECHNIQUE OF PLEURODESIS

Complete pleural fluid evacuation with re-expansion of the underlying lung and apposition of visceral and parietal pleural surfaces is necessary for successful pleurodesis. Adequate fluid drainage is determined by

A

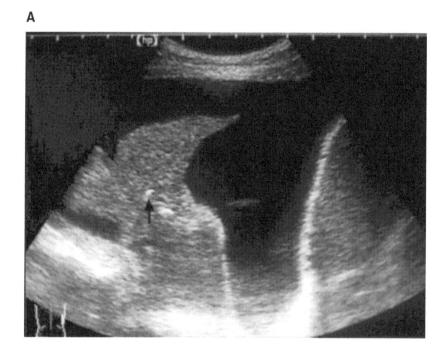

B

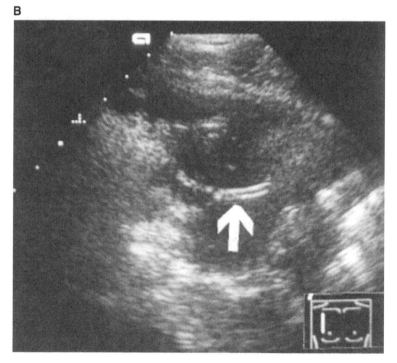

Figure 6
(**A**) Drainage in an echo-free environment is easily recognized. (**B**) Echogenic double reflex of the drainage (*arrow*). *Abbreviations*: D, diaphragm; LU, lung; Pl, pleura; Tu, tumor.

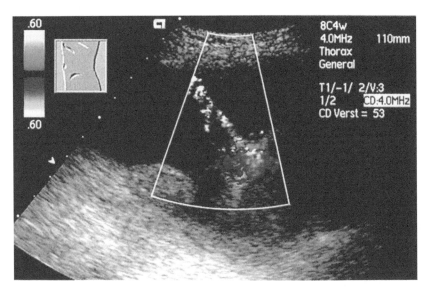

Figure 7
Color Doppler sonography (show here in gray scale). Liquid movement allows detection of needle.

radiographic resolution of the effusion and daily catheter output of less than 100 mL, usually accomplished within five days of drainage catheter placement (48,50,59). A thick pleural peel, endobronchial obstruction, or underlying interstitial lung disease, all of which prevent adequate re-expansion of the lung and obliteration of the pleural space, may preclude successful pleurodesis. Once the effusion has been evacuated and the lung has re-expanded, chemical pleurodesis is performed by intrapleural administration of a sclerosing agent. A variety of agents, including doxycycline, minocycline, bleomycin, *Corynebacterium parvum*, and talc may be used (49,50). Talc, administered as a suspension through a chest tube or insufflated into the pleural space during thoracoscopy, has a success rate of 93% to 95% and is the agent of choice when available (48). Following injection of the sclerosing agent, the catheter is clamped for two hours. The catheter is then reconnected to suction and usually removed the following day (22).

The success of image-guided drainage and sclerosis of malignant effusions is usually defined as absence of symptomatic reaccumulation of fluid one month after sclerosis. Reported success rates of small-bore catheter treatment range from 62% to 92% (1,2,51) and are comparable to those reported with large-bore tubes (52). Procedural complications include infection and self-limited pneumothorax (22,53).

COMPLICATIONS

US-guided drainage is safe and accurate when performed correctly and is associated with a low complication rate (54–59). Chest pain following catheter placement is common (37) and probably results from catheter contact with the parietal pleura. Pneumothorax occurs in 1% of patients, and bleeding or hemoptysis occurs in 0% to 2% of patients (60). Wound infection, chest wall hematoma, and hemothorax may also occur, but are also seen in < 1% of cases. The complication rates of US versus CT guidance are similar (60). There is also a risk of new metastasis in the biopsy channel as a result of the biopsy, and this is particularly true for mesothelioma. In 1995, 95,070 US-guided biopsies were reviewed (61). Six metastases (0.0063%) were detected within the biopsy site after patients underwent fine-needle biopsy. Metastases to the chest wall occurred after large cutting-needle biopsies or after chest tube insertion in 11 cases (0.012%). Metastasis typically occurred with severe and progressive disease. While local metastasis may cause pain, it is not known to decrease life expectancy in patients with carcinoma.

SUMMARY

Sonography is the technique of choice to guide thoracentesis and pleural drainage. Its advantages include absence of ionizing radiation, portability, and real-time capabilities. US is increasingly used to guide interventional procedures of the chest. Percutaneous pleural and lung biopsy can be performed using US guidance, with either the freehand technique or a needle guide. Patients with free-flowing pleural fluid who can sit upright or those with loculated collections that contact the chest wall are easily accessed by sonography. Pleural drainage can also be performed at the bedside using sonographic guidance in critically ill, hemodynamically unstable patients. Complications of image-guided pleural drainage are uncommon but include bleeding due to intercostal vessel injury and pneumothorax.

REFERENCES

1. Herth FJF, Becker HD. Transthoracic ultrasound. Respiration 2003; 70:87–94.
2. Beckh S, Bolcskei P, Lessnau KD. Real-time chest ultrasonography. A comprehensive review for the pulmonologist. Chest 2002; 122:1759–1773.
3. Mathis G. Thorax sonography: part I. Chest wall and pleura. Ultrasound Med Biol 1997; 23:1131–1139.
4. Yang PC, Luh KT, Chang DB, Wu HD, Yu CJ, Kuo SH. Value of sonography in determining the nature of pleural effusion: analysis of 320 cases. Am J Roentgenol 1992; 159:29–33.
5. Shankar S, Gulati M, Kang M, Kang M, Gupta S, Suri S. Image-guided percutaneous drainage of thoracic empyema: can sonography predict the outcome? Eur Radiol 2000; 10:495–499.
6. Reuss J. Sonographic imaging of the pleura: nearly 30 years experience. Eur J Ultrasound 1996; 3:25–39.
7. Gehmacher O, Mathis G, Kopf A, Scheier M. Ultrasound imaging of pneumonia. Ultrasound Med Biol 1995; 21:1119–1122.
8. Yu CJ, Yang PC, Wu HD, Chang DB, Kuo SH, Luh KT. Ultrasound study in unilateral hemithorax opacification: image comparison with CT. Am Rev Respir Dis 1993; 147:430–433.
9. Marel M, Stastny B, Meli nova L, Svandova E, Light RW. Diagnosis of pleural effusions: experience with clinical studies, 1986 to 1990. Chest 1995; 107:1598–1603.
10. Broaddus VC, Light RW. Disorders of the pleura: general principles and diagnostic approach. In: Murray JF, Nadel JA, eds. Textbook of Respiratory Medicine. 2d ed. Philadelphia, PA: WB Saunders, 1994:2156–2160.
11. Mueller PR, Saini S, Simeone JF, Silverman SG, Morris E, Hahn PF, Forman BH, McLoud TC, Shepard JO, Ferrucci JT Jr. Image-guided pleural biopsies: indications, technique, and results in 23 patients. Radiology 1988; 169:1–4.
12. Sniders GL, Saleh SS. Empyema of the thorax inadults: review of 105 cases. Chest 1968; 54:12–17.
13. Light RW. Parapneumonic effusions and empyema. Clin Chest Med 1985; 6:55–62.
14. Strange C, Sahn SA. The clinican's perspective on parapneumonic effusions and empyema. Chest 1993; 103:259–261.
15. Storm HK, Krasnick M, Bang K, Frimodt-Moller N. Treatment of pleural empyema secondary to pneumonia: thoracentesis regimen versus tube drainage. Thorax 1992; 47:821–824.
16. Ramnath RR, Heller RM, Ben-Ami T, Miller MA, Campbell P, Neblett WW III, Holcomb GW, Hernanz-Schulman M. Implications of early sonographic evaluation of parapneumonic effusions in children with pneumonia. Pediatrics 1998; 101:68–71.
17. Shankar KR, Kenny SE, Okoye BO, Carty HM, Lloyd DA, Losty PD. Evolving experience in the management of empyema thoracis. Acta Paediatr 2000; 89:417–420.
18. van Sonnenberg E, D'Agostino HB, Casola G, Wittich GR, Varney RR, Harker C. Lung abscess: CT-guided drainage. Radiology 1991; 178:347–351.
19. Stark DD, Federle MP, Goodman PC, Podrasky AE, Webb WR. Differentiating lung abscess and empyema: radiology and computed tomography. Am J Roentgenol 1983; 141:163–167.
20. Neuhof H, Touroff ASW. Acute putrid abscess of the lung. J Thorac Surg 1942; 12:98–106.
21. Baker RR. The treatment of lung abscess: current concepts. Chest 1985; 87:709–710.
22. Klein JS, Schultz S, Heffner JE. Interventional radiology of the chest: image-guided percutaneous drainage of plerual effusions, lung abscess and pneumothorax. Am J Roentgenol 1995; 164:581–588.

23. Mathis G. Thoraxsonography. II. Peripheral pulmonary consolidation. Ultrasound Med 1997; 23:1141–1153.
24. Yang PC, Luh KT, Lee Chang DB. Ultrasound evaluation of pulmonary consolidation. Am Rev Respir Dis 1992; 146:757–762.
25. Yang PC, Lee YC, Wu HD, Luh KT. Lung tumors associated with obstructive pneumonitis: US studies. Radiology 1990; 174:717–720.
26. Wang HC, Yu CJ, Chang DB, Yuan A, Lee YC, Yang PC, Kuo SH, Luh KT. Transthoracic needle biopsy of thoracic tumors by a color Doppler ultrasound puncture guiding device. Thorax 1995; 50(12):1258–1263.
27. Yang PC. Ultrasound-guided transthoracic biopsy of peripheral lung, pleural, and chest wall lesions. J Thorac Imaging 1997; 12:272–284.
28. Yang PC, Luh KT, Lee YC, Chang DB, Yu CJ, Wu HD, Lee LN, Kuo SH. Lung abcess: ultrasound examination and US-guided transthoracic aspiration. Radiology 1991; 180:171–175.
29. Mueller PR, Berlin L. Complications of lung abscess aspiration and drainage. Am J Roentgenol 2002; 178:1083–1086.
30. Schmitt GS, Ohar JM, Kanter KR, Naunheim KS. Indwelling transbronchial catheter drainage of pulmonary abscess. Ann Thorac Surg 1988; 45:43–47.
31. Ewig S, Schafer H. Treatment of community-acquired lung abscess associated with aspiration. Pneumologie 2001; 55(suppl 9):431–437.
32. Herth F, Ernst A, Becker HD. How to do it: lung abcess drainage. In: Beamis JF, Shapshay S, eds. Proceedings of the 12th World Congress for Bronchology. Bologna: Monduzzi Editore, 2002:99–105.
33. Almind M, Lange P, Viskum K. Spontaneous pneumothorax: comparison of simple drainage, talc pleurodesis, and tetracycline pleurodesis. Thorax 1989; 44:627–630.
34. Conces DJ Jr, Tarver RD, Gray WC, Pearcy EA. Treatment of pneumothoraces utilizing small caliber chest tubes. Chest 1988; 94:55–57.
35. Oaniel TM, Tribble CG, Rodgers BM. Thoracoscopy and talc poudrage for pneumothoraces and effusions. Ann Thorac Surg 1990; 50:186–189.
36. Wu RG, Yang PC, Kuo SH, Luh KT. "Fluid color" sign: a useful indicator for discrimination between pleural thinckening and pleural effusion. J Ultrasound Med 1995; 14:767–769.
37. Minami H, Saka H, Senda K, Horio Y, Iwahara T, Nomura F, Sakai S, Shimokata K. Small caliber catheter drainage for spontaneous pneumothorax. Am J Med Sci 1992; 304:345–347.
38. Casola G, van Sonnenberg E, Keightley A, Ho M, Withers C, Lee AS. Pneumothorax: radiologic treatment with small catheters. Radiology 1988; 166:89–91.
39. Molina PL, Solomon SL, Glazer HS, Sagel SS, Anderson DJ. A one-piece unit for treatment of pneumothorax complicating needle biopsy: evaluation in 10 patients. Am J Roentgenol 1990; 155:31–33.
40. Stavas J, van Sonnenberg E, Casola G, Wittich GR. Percutaneous drainage of infected and noninfected thoracic fluid collections. J Thorac Imaging 1987; 2:80–87.
41. Sheth S, Hamper UM, Stanley DB, Wheeler JH, Smith PA. US guidance for thoracic biopsy: a valuable alternative to CT. Radiology 1999; 210:721–726.
42. Keske U. Ultrasound-aided thoracentesis in intensive care patients. Intensive Care Med 1999; 25:896–897.
43. Tatersall DJ, Traill ZC, Gleeson FV. Chest drains: does size matter? Clin Radiol 2000; 55:415–421.
44. Ulmer JL, Choplin RH, Reed JC. Image-guided catheter drainage of the infected pleural space. J Thorac Imaging 1991; 6:65–73.

45. Robinson LA, Moulton AL, Fleming WH, Alonso A, Galbraith TA. Intrapleural fibrinolytic treatment of multiloculated thoracic empyemas. Ann Thorac Surg 1994; 57:803–814.

46. Moulton JS, Moore PT, Mencini RA. Treatment of loculated pleural effusions with transcatheter intracavitary urokinase. Am J Roentgenol 1989; 153:941–945.

47. Lee KS, Im J-G, Kim YH, Hwang SH, Bae WK, Lee BH. Treatment of thoracic multiloculated empyemas with intracavitary urokinase: a prospective study. Radiology 1991; 179:771–775.

48. Hartman DL, Gaither JM, Kesler KA, Mylet DM, Brown JW, Mathur PN. Comparison of insufflated talc under thoracoscopie guidance with standard tertacycline and bleomycin pleurodesis for control of malignant pleural effusions. J Thorac Cardiovasc Surg 1993; 105:743–748.

49. Walker-Renard PB, Vaughan LM, Sahn SA. Chemical pleurodesis for malignant pleural effusions. Ann Intern Med 1994; 120:56–64.

50. Heffner JE, Standerfer RJ, Torstveit J, Unruh L. Clinical efficacy of doxycyeline for pleurodesis. Chest 1994; 105:1743–1747.

51. Morrison MC, Mueller PR, Lee MJ, Saini S, Brink JA, Dawson SL, Cortell ED, Hahn PF. Sclerotherapy of malignant pleural effusions through sonographically placed small-bore catheters. Am J Roentgenol 1992; 158:41–43.

52. Ruckdeschel JC, Moores D, Lee JY, Einhorn LH, Mandelbaum I, Koeller J, Weiss GR, Losada M, Keller JH. Intrapleural therapy for malignant pleural effusions: a randomized comparison of bleomycin and tetracycline. Chest 1991; 100:1528–1535.

53. Goff BA, Mueller PR, Muntz HG, Rice LW. Small chest-tube drainage followed by bleomycin sclerosis for malignant pleural effusions. Obstet Gynecol 1993; 8:993–996.

54. Pope TL Jr. Percutaneous needle biopsy and percutaneous empyema drainage. In: Armstrong P, Wilson AG, Dee P, eds. Imaging of Diseases of the Chest. St. Louis, MO: Mosby, 1990:881–886.

55. Chang DB, Yang PC, Luh KT, Kuo SH, Yu CJ. Ultrasound-guided pleural biopsy with Tru-Cut needle. Chest 1991; 100:1328–1333.

56. Hsu WH, Chiang CD, Hsu JY, Kwan PC, Chen CL, Chen CY. Ultrasound-guided aspiration biopsy of anterior mediastinal masses. J Clin Ultrasound 1991; 19:209–214.

57. Yuan A, Yang PC, Chang DB, Yu CJ, Lee YC, Kuo SH, Luh KT. Ultrasound-guided aspiration biopsy of small peripheral pulmonary nodules. Chest 1992; 101:926–930.

58. Pan JF, Yang PC, Chang DB, Lee YC, Kuo SH, Luh KT. Needle aspiration biopsy of malignant lung masses with necrotic centers. Chest 1993; 103:1452–1456.

59. Sheth S, Hamper UM, Stanley DB, Wheeler JH, Smith PA. US guidance for thoracic biopsy: a valuable alternative to CT. Radiology 1999; 210:721–726.

60. Beckh S, Bölcskei PL. Biopsy of thoracic lesions: from CT-controlled to ultrasound guidance. Ultraschall Med 1997; 18:220–225.

61. Weiss H, Duntsch U. Complications of fine-needle puncture. Ultraschall Med 1996; 17:118–130.

5

Ultrasound-Guided Transthoracic Needle Biopsy

Peter Doelken
Division of Pulmonary and Critical Care Medicine, Allergy and Clinical Immunology Medical University of South Carolina, Charleston, South Carolina, U.S.A.

INTRODUCTION

Ultrasound (US)-guided transthoracic needle biopsy is an underutilized technique with an excellent safety record. US-guided biopsy is especially suitable for peripheral lung lesions and some anterior mediastinal masses, both of which are frequently beyond the reach of bronchoscopic biopsy techniques. Thus, US-guided transthoracic needle biopsy complements the biopsy techniques available to the bronchoscopist. US-guided needle biopsy of chest lesions is not only a viable alternative to computed tomography (CT) guidance but is the preferable modality in many cases. Provided the lesion can be visualized with US, biopsy can be performed faster and does not require the patient to remain in a certain position for prolonged periods of time. In addition, there is no radiation exposure. Lung lesions abutting the visceral pleura are easily visualized with US, as are pleural masses, pleural thickening, and some anterior mediastinal masses (Figs. 1 and 2) (1–7).

Basic requirements for the safe and successful practice of US-guided transthoracic needle biopsy include a cooperative patient, the availability of appropriate equipment, and proficiency in the field of chest ultrasonography. Fortunately, apart from disposable biopsy needles, no additional expensive equipment, such as transducers with integrated needle guide, are required for transthoracic interventions. When available, however, dedicated biopsy transducers may be used to facilitate biopsy in some cases.

Operator proficiency in chest sonography, on the other hand, is critical. The pulmonologist must be familiar with all aspects of transthoracic pleural and pulmonary US, and must be able to correlate CT images of

A

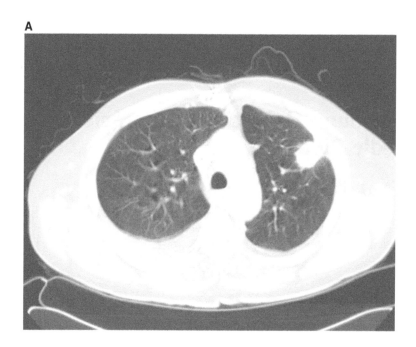

B

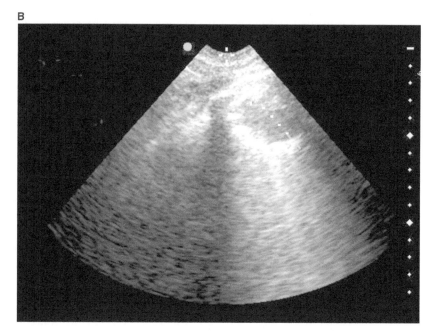

Figure 1
(**A**) The CT shows a mass slightly larger than 3 cm in the left upper lobe. The lesion abuts the chest wall in the area of an intercostal space. (**B**) The corresponding US image shows the mass and rib shadows at left and right. The depth and size of the lesion are marked. The biopsy was performed without real-time imaging and the diagnosis of metastatic non-small cell lung cancer was made on site. *Abbreviations*: US, ultrasound; CT, computed tomography.

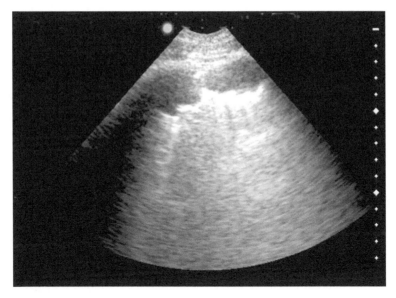

Figure 2
This US image shows anechoic subpleural metastases of an angiosarcoma.
The nodules were not sampled because the diagnosis was ascertained by other
means. The lesions would be excellent targets for US-guided biopsy. Core
biopsy in all likelihood would be necessary because of the type of malignancy.
Abbreviation: US, ultrasound.

the chest with US findings. The details of diagnostic transthoracic chest
sonography are reviewed elsewhere in this volume and are beyond the
scope of this chapter. The biopsy techniques described here are not
technically difficult but should only be attempted by pulmonologists
performing chest US at expert level (8–18).

Any review of percutaneous transthoracic needle biopsy is in
part subjective, due to the particular techniques a practitioner may
utilize. This chapter discusses only the coaxial biopsy technique because
that is this author's expertice. Coaxial technique utilizes an introducer
cannula with a stylet, which is removed after placement, and all biopsies
are obtained through the lumen of the introducer. This author believes
that coaxial techniques are best suited for the purpose, of course others
may disagree. Special biopsy transducers are not used because of the cost
versus benefit ratio. In the end, one must make a decision for or against
a specific technical variation based on personal preference, training
background, and resource availability.

ULTRASOUND EQUIPMENT

Chest US should be performed with convex array transducers with a
frequency range of 2 to 5 MHz. The convex shape of these transducers

facilitates scanning through the intercostal spaces. An important consideration in the choice of equipment is the quality of near-field imaging because of the superficial location of some lesions. In the thin individual, poor near-field resolution may result in an inability to image small lesions. The same transducers may be used for US-guided transthoracic biopsy. Dedicated interventional transducers with needle guide or snap-on needle guides are not required. The procedure is performed under sterile conditions and a sterile transducer sleeve may be used to maintain sterility (8,11,12).

IMAGING

US is not suitable for general diagnostic imaging of the chest because of the limited views available. CT is usually necessary to localize and demonstrate the extent of intrathoracic pathology, prior to an intervention. Once lesions suitable for US-guided biopsy are identified, US should be performed to further characterize the lesions. The prerequisite for US-guided biopsy is the presence of a US window, that is the absence of bone or air overlying the biopsy target. Obviously, vital structures may not lie within the biopsy needle path. With these criteria satisfied, US will add diagnostic information to CT-imaging through its superior ability to distinguish solid tissue from fluid and consolidated lung. This ability is particularly advantageous if partially necrotic lung lesions or mass lesions of the pleura in the presence of pleural fluid are targeted. In these cases, the US-guided biopsy may be directed to the solid areas with higher success rate than CT-guided biopsy. Once the target is identified, the surrounding structures are identified. With a safe biopsy path identified, entry angle and depth are determined. After needle insertion at the appropriate angle and depth, US may be used to confirm needle position. If real-time visualization of the biopsy needle is desired, when using the free hand technique, care must be taken to correctly identify the needle tip. This is best accomplished by keeping the needle path parallel to the scanning plane and then applying small corrections at 90° to the scanning plane until the needle is visualized. The most common cause for failure to visualize the needle is inadvertent angulation of the scanning plane with respect to the needle path, resulting in an oblique intersection of the scanning plane and needle path or needle. The coordination skills required for successful application of the free hand technique may be practiced with homemade models consisting of gelatin and fruits. Alternatively, one may practice routine real-time visualization during drainage catheter insertion into large pleural effusions. The skills so acquired will easily transfer to transthoracic needle biopsy. Transducers with built-in needle guides do not allow the needle to deviate from the scanning plane and therefore require less skill during real-time image guidance but may be more cumbersome to use (11–13,19,20).

FINE NEEDLE ASPIRATION

Fine needle aspiration can be performed with 21 gauge or smaller spinal needles attached to a 10 cc syringe. Microscopy slides and preservation media need to be available. After localizing the target lesion, local anesthesia is given and the depth and angle of needle insertion are determined. An 18 or 20 gauge introducer needle with a removable stylet is then inserted through a small skin incision to the appropriate depth, with or without real-time guidance. Introducers of this type are part of some disposable automatic tissue sampling kits such as the Temno Evolution™ (Cardinal Health, Ohio, U.S.). Patients are asked to hold their breath while the needle is advanced, whenever the introducer is not occluded and also during the actual biopsy. If the target lesion is in the lung, the needle will move slightly with the respiratory cycle when positioned in the lung, unless the lung is adherent to the parietal pleura. Oftentimes, some resistance is encountered when a lesion is entered, indicating proper placement. The stylet is then removed from the introducer and the needle is inserted. Once the needle is advanced to the appropriate depth, suction is applied and the needle is moved back and forth several times while maintaining suction. Suction is then discontinued and the needle removed. Suction should not be applied during insertion and withdrawal of the needle to prevent dilution of the sample. Slides may be immediately assessed for adequacy by on-site cytopathology.

Repeat biopsies may be taken from different areas by slightly changing the angle of the introducer. The use of an introducer allows these repeat biopsies without additional punctures of the pleura. The primary advantage of fine needle aspiration is safety due to the small size of the needle. A disadvantage, however, is the small amount of specimen obtained. Histologic diagnosis is rarely possible and the tumor type often cannot be determined with the cytopathology alone. At any time, a cutting needle may be advanced through the introducer to obtain a core sample, if on-site cytopathology indicates inadequate material (21–24).

CORE NEEDLE BIOPSY

Spring-activated cutting needle biopsy kits are available from several manufacturers. Sizes 18 to 20 gauge are sufficient for most work. Most automatic side-cutting needles have a fixed throw and consequently a biopsy channel of approximately 20 mm. Adjustable throw needles are also available and may be advantageous for smaller lesions or lesions in proximity to vital structures. The insertion procedure is similar to the fine needle aspiration. Again, patients are asked to hold their breath while the needle is advanced, whenever the introducer is not occluded, and also during the actual biopsy. After removal of the stylet from the introducer, the activated cutting needle is inserted and immediately discharged. I orient the cutting apparatus caudally to minimize the risk of injury to intercostal vessels and nerves, when performing biopsies close to the pleura. The beveled tip of the cutting apparatus of an automatic sampling system may cause the needle to describe a curved path during firing, if resistance is encountered. It is therefore important to consider this possible deviation from the straight path. The sloped side of the needle should be facing any structure at risk for injury. The needle will then describe a path away from the structure if it should deviate from a straight line (9). The obtained biopsies are rolled across a microscopic slide and then transferred into an appropriate medium. The slides can be immediately assessed for adequacy. The procedure may be repeated several times. The advantage of core biopsy is the amount of tissue obtained, allowing histologic diagnosis in a large percentage of cases. It also appears to be a safe technique with a very low complication rate of 1.8% in a series of 218 patients with lesions 3 cm or larger (6,21–24).

LUNG

Any lesion visible with US may be a target for US-guided biopsy. Indications for US-guided biopsy are similar to the indications for CT-guided biopsy. Mass lesions with fluid-filled necrotic centers are preferably accessed with US-guidance, with the superior ability of US to distinguish solids from liquids (Fig. 3) (25). Lesions containing air may be better visualized by CT-guided biopsy, and US-guided biopsy needs to be considered on a case-by-case basis. Accessible lesions can be diagnosed with a high degree of accuracy, and even nodules < 3 cm in diameter may be accessed successfully. Successful diagnosis of malignancy can be expected in up to 97% cases when core biopsy is performed. Fine needle aspiration is also suitable for diagnosis of lung malignancy, although determination of the specific type of tumor, with the exception of small cell lung cancer, may require acquisition of core biopsies (6). The sensitivity of fine needle aspiration for malignancy is approximately 80% and this provides the rationale to perform needle aspiration prior to core biopsy, provided on-site cytopathology is available. For example, a positive cytology is often all what is needed to document metastasis. In these cases, core needle biopsy may be omitted, lowering the already small risk of percutaneous transthoracic needle biopsy even further. If on-site cytopathology is not available, core biopsy should be performed in almost all cases. In cases where a benign cause for the lesion is suspected, core biopsies need to be obtained and specimens should be sent for the appropriate microbiologic tests. Chronic cavitating or bronchiectatic lesions are not good candidates for percutaneous core biopsy due to the increased risk of bleeding. These lesions are often highly vascularized and arterial bleeds may be precipitated. However, these cases need to be considered on an individual basis and US-guided biopsy may still emerge as the best option in selected cases (1,3,5,7,14,21–24). Occasionally, lung abscesses fail to respond to conservative therapy and drainage becomes necessary. US-guidance can be used for diagnostic and therapeutic aspiration or drainage catheter placement. Lung abscesses may only be separated from

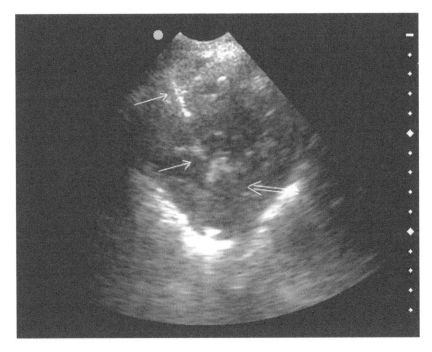

Figure 3
This still image of a real-time US-guided core biopsy depicts the needle and its tip (*arrows*), just prior to deployment of the cutting apparatus. The needle is positioned in a cavity filled with fluid and debris. The target is the thick posterior wall of the lesion (*double arrow*). Material suspicious for malignancy was obtained, while a prior CT-guided biopsy attempt only obtained pus. A necrotizing adenocarcinoma was found at surgery. *Abbreviations*: US, ultrasound; CT, computed tomography.

the pleura by a rim of consolidated lung providing an acceptable sonographic window (26,27).

PLEURA

Metastatic disease of the pleura is commonly diagnosed by pleural fluid cytology, and simple fluid aspiration is the appropriate initial test if malignant pleural effusion is suspected. In cases where fluid cytology is inconclusive, US-guided pleural biopsy may be performed. US allows selection of abnormal areas of the parietal pleura for biopsy; presumably, the yield of targeted biopsy exceeds the yield of random sampling of the pleura (24,27). Standard coaxial cutting needles may be used for pleural biopsy; Cope or Abrams needles are also suitable. Try to orient the needle in such a way that the cutting apparatus is directed caudally to minimize the risk of injury to the intercostal vessels. As this is also the sloped side of the needle, any needle tip deflection when resistance is encountered will be cranial, which is advantageous when working close to the diaphragm.

Obviously, needle orientation may have to be modified if vital structures are in the path of possible needle deviation (19,20,28,29).

Malignant pleural mesothelioma cannot be diagnosed with cytology alone, and good quality tissue samples need to be obtained. The costophrenic recess is often a good target area and the frequent presence of pleural fluid simplifies the task. The biopsy specimens should be macroscopically examined. Homogeneous tissue cylinders indicate viable tumor tissue, whereas fragmented bloody specimens may signify necrosis or fibrin. Several good quality specimens should be obtained. US-guided biopsy should probably be considered the initial procedure of choice in the evaluation of pleural mesothelioma. The simplicity and low cost of the procedure coupled with an acceptable sensitivity of 77% and a specificity of 88%, in one small series, are arguments in favor of such an approach (30,31).

MEDIASTINUM

The anterior mediastinum is usually inaccessible to US imaging due to obscuration by overlying bone or aerated lung. Anterior mediastinal masses can displace the adjacent lung and become excellent targets for US-guided percutaneous biopsy. The operator must have a thorough understanding of the local anatomy and must be expert in accurate needle placement. Attempts at biopsy with needle aspiration only, in order to increase safety, are ill-advised in the anterior mediastinum. The diagnostic yield of cytology alone is too low to justify the procedure. Essentially, except in cases where carcinoma is highly suspected, core biopsies must be obtained. Accurate diagnosis of common malignant anterior mediastinal masses, such as thymoma, lymphoma, and some germ cell tumors, as well as benign disease, requires histologic specimens (2,7,15,16).

CONTRAINDICATIONS

There are few absolute contraindications to percutaneous transthoracic biopsy. The most important absolute contraindications are an uncooperative patient, a patient who cannot be maintained in the optimal position for biopsy, and intractable coughing. All other contraindications are relative and need a judicious evaluation of the risk of biopsy and the alternatives. Severe coagulopathies, thrombocytopenia of < 50,000, and uremic platelet dysfunction are also considered contraindications in my practice, unless corrected prior to the procedure. Routine laboratory evaluation of prothrombin time (PT) and partial thromboplastin time (PTT) or platelets in patients who have no history of bleeding problems and who are not taking anticoagulants are probably not indicated and these tests should be reserved for patients at risk for bleeding due to underlying disease. Patients with severe underlying lung disease or with a single lung will require immediate treatment for pneumothorax, and preparations should be made prior to biopsy. The author does not perform percutaneous lung biopsies in mechanically ventilated patients but would certainly consider pleural biopsy and mediastinal biopsy on a case-by-case basis. In any case, consideration of percutaneous transthoracic biopsy in the critically ill should be extremely uncommon. Severe pulmonary hypertension a relative contraindication, should also be considered for percutaneous lung biopsy (8–10,17,18).

COMPLICATIONS

Transthoracic US-guided biopsy has a low complication rate in expert hands. With the exception of air embolism, the complications encountered are similar to the complications of transbronchial biopsy, and pulmonologists are familiar with their management. The pneumothorax rate associated with biopsy of lung lesions is approximately 3% (1,3–7,11,21). Most patients develop some pleuritic chest pain when pneumothorax occurs. Due to this low rate of pneumothorax and the fact that some of the reported cases were of minimal size and did not require treatment, routine postprocedure chest radiographs in the asymptomatic patient with unchanged physical examination are probably not cost effective. The decision to obtain a chest radiograph after the procedure should be made on a case-by-case basis. If US is used for image guidance, even minimal pneumothoraces will lead to an immediate loss of imaging capability and the procedure must be terminated. This fact is also the only disadvantage of US-guidance when compared with CT-guidance. CT-guided biopsy can proceed even in the presence of a pneumothorax and CT allows assessment of the size of a pneumothorax. Although US-guided biopsy of lung lesions has a lower overall rate of pneumothorax than CT-guided biopsy, this difference is due to restriction of US-guided biopsy to lesions abutting the pleura where the needle does not need to pass through aerated lung. Pneumothorax rates for CT-guided and US-guided biopsies are not different when intraparenchymal lesions not amenable to US-guided biopsy are excluded from the analysis. The rate of pneumothorax may be further decreased by positioning the patient on the biopsy site and by limiting activity for some time after the procedure. Not all pneumothoraces require thoracotomy tube placement. Small pneumothoraces causing only minimal symptoms may be followed by observation. In other cases simple aspiration may suffice. If thoracostomy tube placement is required, outpatient treatment with a small bore catheter attached to a Heimlich valve is an acceptable option. Commercial kits incorporating catheter and valve in one device are available, which reduces the risk of accidental disconnection and eliminates the problem of accidentally connecting the Heimlich valve incorrectly.

Hemoptysis may occur in up to 10% of cases when core biopsy is performed (14). It is usually minimal and no cause for concern. Massive hemoptysis does occur and is associated with an increased mortality. It is fortunately rare and is managed similarly to hemoptysis from transbrochial biopsy. As the site of bleeding is known, tamponade with a bronchoscope, balloon tamponade, and selective intubation of the contralateral side may all be employed to stabilize the patient until definitive therapy can be administered. Pulmonologists are likely to perform US-guided biopsies in the bronchoscopy suite, and they are, due to their expertise in fiber optic bronchoscopy, in an excellent position to manage this rare but dangerous complication. Hemoptysis may cause severe coughing due to irritation of the bronchi. If severe coughing occurs, the introducer needs to be withdrawn to prevent tearing of the pleura, and introduction of air into pulmonary veins or venules could happen if the introducer happens to be located in these vessels. Coughing-related large intrathoracic pressure swings could lead to introduction of significant amounts of air into the pulmonary veins with the consequence of systemic air embolism.

Even without coughing, air embolism may occur. Due to the location of US-accessible lesions in the lung periphery, away from large pulmonary veins, the risk of this complication is likely lower than in CT-guided biopsies of central lesions. The risk may be further reduced by occluding the introducer cannula with the stylet between needle passes and by repositioning the transducer when excessive amounts of blood are encountered. If air embolism occurs, the patient should be placed in the left lateral decubitus position and 100% oxygen administered; hyperbaric oxygen therapy should be considered if available. It should be mentioned that inadvertent puncture of vital organs, such as the heart or major vessels, may occur due to inadequate technique. This type of complication is likely related to operator proficiency and should be avoidable by the expert (10,32–34).

CONCLUSION

US-guided percutaneous transthoracic needle biopsy is a modality with an excellent safety record and a diagnostic accuracy equal to or exceeding the accuracy of CT-guided biopsy. It is the modality of choice for lesions visible with US. Pulmonologists with experience in chest US will find the technique to be an excellent addition to their interventional practice. Pulmonologists are familiar with the recognition and treatment of the possible complications and can perform the procedure in the bronchoscopy procedure suite. With pulmonary fellowship programs increasingly incorporating sonography into their clinical curriculum, future graduates will be in an excellent position to make percutaneous transthoracic needle biopsy part of their practice.

REFERENCES

1. Yuan A, Yang P-C, Chan D-B, Yu CJ, Lee YC, Kuo SH, Luh KT. Ultrasound-guided aspiration biopsy of small peripheral pulmonary nodules. Chest 1992; 101:926–930.
2. Yu C-J, Yang P-C, Chang D-B, Wu HD, Lee LN, Lee YC, Kuo SH, Luh KT. Evaluation of ultrasonically guided biopsies of mediastinal masses. Chest 1992; 100:399–405.
3. Yang P-C, Luh K-T, Sheu J-C, Kuo SH, Yang SP. Peripheral pulmonary lesions: ultrasonography and ultrasonically guided aspiration biopsy. Radiology 1985; 155:451–456.
4. Sheth S, Hamper UM, Stanley DB, Wheeler JH, Smith PA. US guidance for thoracic biopsy: a valuable alternative to CT. Radiology 1999; 210:721–726.
5. Ikezoe J, Morimoto S, Arisawa J, Takashima S, Kozuka T, Nakahara K. Percutaneous biopsy of thoracic lesions: value of sonography for needle guidance. Am J Roentgenol 1990; 154:1181–1185.
6. Yang P-C, Chang D-B, Yu C-J, Lee YC, Wu HD, Kuo SH, Luh KT. Ultrasound-guided core biopsy of thoracic tumors. Am Rev Respir Dis 1992; 146:763–767.
7. Pedersen OM, Aasen TB, Gulsvik A. Fine needle aspiration biopsy of mediastinal and peripheral pulmonary masses guided by real-time sonography. Chest 1986; 89:504–508.
8. Charboneau JW, Reading CC, Welch TJ. CT and sonographically guided needle biopsy: current techniques and new innovations. Am J Roentgenol 1990; 154:1–10.
9. Heilo A. US-guided transthoracic biopsy. Eur J Ultrasound 1996; 3:141–151.
10. Moore EH. Technical aspects of needle aspiration lung biopsy: a personal perspective. Radiology 1998; 208:303–318.
11. Bekh S, Boelcskei PL. Biopsie thorakaler Raumforderungen – Von der computertomographischen zur ultraschallgezielten Punktion. Ultraschall Med 1997; 18:220–225.
12. Matalon TAS, Bruce S. US guidance of interventional procedures. Radiology 1990; 174:43–47.
13. Bekh S, Boelcskei PL, Lessnau K-D. Real-time chest ultrasonography. A comprehensive review for the pulmonologist. Chest 2002; 122:1759–1773.
14. Lucidarme O, Howarth N, Finet JF, Grenier PA. Intrapulmonary lesions: percutaneous automatedbiopsy with a detachable, 18-gauge, coaxial cutting needle. Radiology 1998; 207:759–765.
15. Wernecke K, Vassallo P, Peters PE, von Bassewitz DB. Mediastinal tumors: biopsy under US guidance. Radiology 1989; 172:473–476.
16. Saito T, Kobayashi H, Sugama Y, Tamaki S, Kawai T, Kitamura S. Ultrasonically guided needle biopsy in the diagnosis of mediastinal masses. Am Rev Resp Dis 1988; 138:679–684.
17. Klein JS. Interventional techniques in the thorax. Clin Chest Med 1999; 20:805–826.
18. Weisbrod GL. Transthoracic percutaneous lung biopsy. Radiol Clin North Am 1990; 28(3):647–655.
19. Reuss J. Sonographic imaging of the pleura: nearly 30 years experience. Eur J Ultrasound 1996; 3:125–139.
20. Dubs-Kunz B. Sonography of the chest wall. Eur J Ultrasound 1996; 3:103–111.
21. Yang P-C, Lee YC, Yu C-J, Wu HD, Lee LN, Kuo SH, Luh KT. Ultrasonographically guided biopsy of thoracic tumors: a comparison of large-bore cutting biopsy with fine-needle aspiration. Cancer 1992; 69:2553–2560.
22. McLoud TC. Should cutting needles replace needle aspiration of lung lesions? Radiology 1998; 208:269–570.
23. Weiss H, Duentsch U. Komplikationen der Feinnadelpunktion. DEGUM-Umfrage II. Ultraschall in Med 1996; 17:118–130.
24. Chang D-B, Yang P-C, Luh K-T, Kuo SH, Yu CJ. Ultrasound-guided pleural biopsy with Tru-Cut needle. Chest 1991; 100:1328–1333.

25. Pan J-F, Yang P-C, Chang D-B, Lee Y-C, Kuo SH, Luh KT. Needle aspiration biopsy of malignant lung masses with necrotic centers: improved sensitivity with ultrasonic guidance. Chest 1993; 103:1452–1456.
26. Yang P-C, Luh K-T, Lee Y-C, Chang DB, Yu CJ, Wu HD, Lee LN, Kuo SH. Lung abscesses: US examination and US-guided aspiration. Radiology 1991; 180:171–175.
27. Van Sonnenberg E, D'Agostino HB, Casola G, Wittich GR, Varney RR, Harker C. Lung abscess: CT-guided drainage. Radiology 1991; 178:347–351.
28. Mueller PR, Saini S, Simeone JF, Silverman SG, Morris E, Hahn PF, Forman BH, McLoud TC, Shepard JO, Ferrucci JT Jr. Image-guided pleural biopsies: indications, technique and results in 23 patients. Radiology 1988; 169:1–4.
29. O'Moore PV, Mueller PR, Simeone JF, Saini S, Butch RJ, Hahn PF, Steiner E, Stark DD, Ferrucci JT Jr. Sonographic guidance in diagnostic and therapeutic interventions in the pleural space. Am J Roentgenol 1987; 149:1–5.
30. Layer G, Schmitteckert H, Steudel A, Tuengerthal S, Schirren J, van Kaick G, Schild HH. MRT, CT und Sonographie in der praeoperativen Beurteilung der Primaertumorausdehnung beim malignen Pleuramesotheliom. Fortschr Roentgenstr 1999; 170:365–370.
31. Heilo A, Stenwig AE, Solheim OP. Malignant pleural mesothelioma: US-guide histologic core-needle biopsy. Radiology 1999; 211:657–659.
32. Moore EH, Shepard JA, McLoud TC, Templeton PA, Kosiuk JP. Positional precautions in needle aspiration lung biopsy. Radiology 1990; 175:733–735.
33. Brown KT, Brody LA, Getrajdman GI, Napp TE. Outpatient treatment of iatrogenic pneumothorax after needle biopsy. Radiology 1997; 205:249–252.
34. Yankelevitz DF, Davis SD, Henschke CI. Aspiration of a large pneumothorax resulting from transthoracic needle biopsy. Radiology 1996; 200:695–697.

6

The Use of Ultrasound in Trauma

Carlo L. Rosen
Beth Israel Deaconess Medical Center, Harvard Affiliated Emergency Medicine Residency, Boston, Massachusetts, U.S.A.
and Harvard Medical School, Boston, Massachusetts, U.S.A.

Carrie D. Tibbles
Beth Israel Deaconess Medical Center, Harvard Affiliated Emergency Medicine Residency, Boston, Massachusetts, U.S.A.

Jason A. Tracy
Beth Israel Deaconess Medical Center, Harvard Affiliated Emergency Medicine Residency, Boston, Massachusetts, U.S.A.

INTRODUCTION

Ultrasonography of the trauma patient has its roots in Japan and Germany where it has been used for years as part of the initial assessment of the trauma patient (1,2). Recently, in the United States, ultrasonography has become an integral part of trauma resuscitation. In fact, ultrasonography has become part of the American College of Surgeons' Advanced Trauma Life Support guidelines as a diagnostic tool for detecting hemoperitoneum (3). The trauma examination is referred to as the FAST examination—Focused Assessment with Sonography for Trauma. It is currently used in the majority of trauma centers in the United States for the initial evaluation of patients with blunt and penetrating trauma (4). Ultrasound (US) should be part of the secondary survey of the trauma patient. It is a triage tool that helps the resuscitation team decide whether the unstable blunt trauma patient should go directly to the operating room or to the radiology suite for computerized tomography (CT) scan or angiography. For these patients, ultrasonography has replaced diagnostic peritoneal lavage (DPL). In the patient with penetrating trauma, ultrasonography can rapidly detect pericardial effusion and tamponade as an indicator of cardiac injury. Ultrasonography is also used to detect hemothorax. In a clinical situation where minutes count, ultrasonography decreases the time to operative intervention in the trauma patient. In addition, it facilitates the rapid performance of life-saving procedures such as tube thoracostomy.

ADVANTAGES AND DISADVANTAGES

Bedside ultrasonography is perfectly suited for the trauma setting. The examination itself can be performed in two to three minutes (5). Compared with other types of ultrasonography examinations, such as the biliary tract examination, the trauma examination is technically simple and easy. The proportion of indeterminate or uninterpretable examinations is reported to be < 7% (6). The main advantage of the test is that it is portable, and can be repeated easily as necessary. In this respect, ultrasonography is truly an extension of the physical examination. If the clinical status of the patient deteriorates, the examination can be repeated in the trauma room (7). Performance of the test does not require moving the patient out of the resuscitation room where monitoring capabilities are optimal. The performance of serial examinations has also been shown to increase the sensitivity of the test (8). It is recommended that the examination be repeated after half an hour and at regular intervals while the patient is being observed in the emergency department. This technique increases the likelihood of detecting ongoing hemorrhage. Because of the safety of ultrasonography compared with CT, this is an optimal study for detecting intraperitoneal bleeding in the pregnant trauma patient.

As with any diagnostic test, it is critical to know the limitations or disadvantages of the test. US does not define the organ that is injured. The primary goal is to detect the presence or absence of hemoperitoneum as an indicator of intraperitoneal injury. It is not accurate for detecting specific injuries. Because ultrasonography cannot be used to grade or detect specific injuries, it does not replace the use of CT scan in the work-up of trauma patients.

It primarily has limitations in detecting bleeding < 250 cc. Thus, even solid organ injuries with small amounts of hemorrhage will be missed. In addition, hollow viscous, mesenteric, and diaphragmatic injuries, which are usually associated with minimal bleeding, will not be detected (9–11). A negative ultrasonography does not rule out an injury. Finally, the retroperitoneal space is hard to visualize with ultrasonography, making the test insensitive for detecting retroperitoneal bleeding.

INDICATIONS

The true indication for ultrasonography in the trauma setting is the presence of a patient with a history of trauma and an ultrasound machine in the same resuscitation area. Although ultrasonography is primarily utilized for decision-making in unstable blunt trauma patients, it is indicated for all blunt trauma patients as part of the secondary survey regardless of their stability. In the hypotensive blunt trauma patient, the ultrasonography results become the primary branch point for management. Patients with a positive ultrasonography require immediate laparotomy, whereas those with negative FAST examinations require investigation and management for other causes of hypotension. This may include angiography in the case of major pelvic fractures to assess the retroperitoneal bleeding and facilitate embolization of bleeding vessels.

Another indication for the FAST examination in the unstable blunt trauma patient is for the detection of hemothorax. Performing the ultrasonography examination takes less time than waiting for the plain chest radiograph to be developed.

In the stable blunt trauma patient, ultrasonography should not replace CT for the reasons discussed above. However, there are valid reasons for performing the FAST examination in these patients. Even if the resuscitation team has made the decision to perform abdominal CT scan based on mechanism or abdominal tenderness, the ultrasound result determines the speed with which the CT must be performed and provides vital information to the physicians. If the ultrasound is positive for hemoperitoneum, then the patient should undergo CT scan immediately to define the injury. If the patient becomes unstable at any time during the emergency department course, then emergent laparotomy is indicated. If the initial ultrasound is negative for hemoperitoneum, the CT can be done on an urgent, but not emergent, basis.

Patients with penetrating abdominal trauma should undergo the FAST examination to detect intraperitoneal hemorrhage. Obviously, these patients will still need further work-up if the ultrasonography examination is negative. However, if positive, the ultrasonography can result in an immediate decision to proceed to the operating room. As US can rapidly and accurately detect pericardial effusion, all patients with penetrating chest trauma should have an ultrasound examination of the heart and pericardium (12–14).

TECHNIQUE AND FINDINGS

The FAST examination is performed with the patient in the supine position. The four standard views are obtained with the 3.5 MHz probe in the right-upper quadrant, subxiphoid, left-upper quadrant, and suprapubic locations (Fig. 1). Some authors include views of the paracolic gutters; however, these additional views add little diagnostic information and take additional time to perform.

The goal of the FAST examination is to visualize intraperitoneal fluid in dependant areas of the abdominal cavity. Initial fluoroscopy research found that fluid within the abdomen is most likely to accumulate in the suprapubic rectovesicular (male) and rectouterine (female) spaces. Fluid from the upper abdomen travels down the right paracolic gutter to collect suprapubically. Since the phrenocolic ligament prevents the spread of fluid down the left paracolic gutter, fluid from the left-upper quadrant spills over to the right-upper quadrant (Morison's pouch), making this the most dependent area in the upper abdomen (15).

The first and easiest view to obtain is of the right-upper quadrant hepatorenal space, also known as Morison's pouch. The probe is placed in the right mid-axillary line in the longitudinal axis with the probe

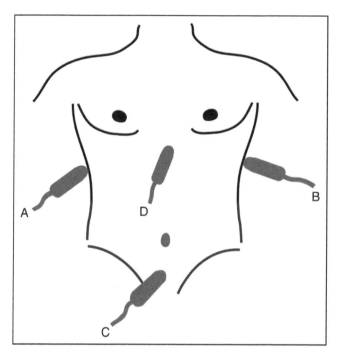

Figure 1
FAST Exam Probe Positions: Morison's pouch (A), splenorenal space (B), suprapubic view (C), and subcoastal veiw (D).

indicator pointing cephalad (Fig. 2). With the probe in the 8th through 11th rib interspace, an initial view of the right kidney helps guide optimal visualization of the interface between the liver and kidney (Morison's pouch). If the view is obscured by a rib, the probe can be angled towards the transverse plane therefore allowing the beam to pass between the ribs. A sweeping motion of the probe beam in the anterior/posterior and cephalad/caudad directions can also bring the kidney into view as well as provide complete visualization of Morison's pouch.

If there is difficulty in finding Morison's pouch, the probe should be moved to a different interspace, with similar sweeping motions of the probe applied to the new location. Since the kidney is a retroperitoneal structure, it is important to place the probe far enough posterior in the axillary line. Having the patient take a deep breath will move the liver and Morison's pouch into view by inflating the lung.

Intraperitoneal blood is anechoic (black) on ultrasonography. In the right-upper quadrant view, this appears as a stripe of black fluid between the liver and the hyperechoic (white) Gerota's fascia which surrounds the kidney (Fig. 3). It is important to remember that any intraperitoneal fluid (i.e., ascites, urine, and bile) appears anechoic making it necessary to incorporate the clinical situation into ultrasonography interpretation. Further difficulty can arise when visualizing the kidneys,

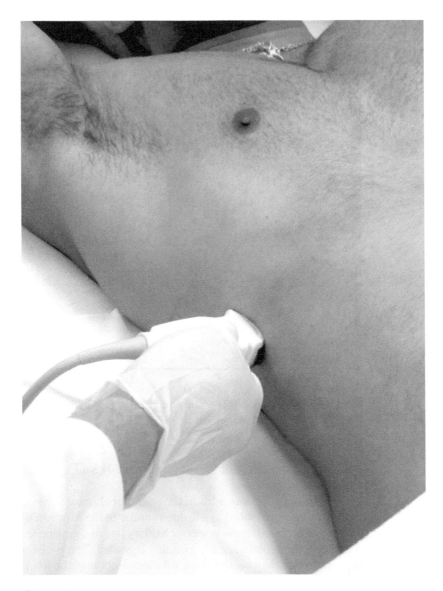

Figure 2
Probe position for Morison's Pouch view.

especially in obese patients, as perinephric fat can sometimes be confused with fluid in Morison's pouch.

The liver and renal parenchyma may be fully visualized for hematomas. These will appear as anechoic or hyperechoic areas within the organs. This can, however, be technically difficult as ultrasonography has a low sensitivity for detecting parenchymal injury even in experienced hands. Imaging of the right-upper quadrant is complete once the hyperechoic diaphragm and right thorax are examined for a hemothorax. As

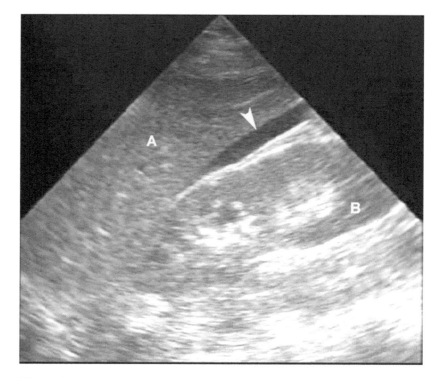

Figure 3
Fluid in Morison's Pouch. The arrow represents fluid in the space between the liver (A) and the right kidney (B).

discussed below, ultrasonography can reliably and quickly locate fluid within the thorax.

In the left-upper quadrant, the splenorenal space is viewed next. The examination is performed in a fashion similar to the Morison's pouch view. The probe is placed in the posterior axillary line at the same level as on the right, with the probe indicator pointing cephalad. The probe will likely be more posterior than on the right, with localization of the left kidney being more difficult due to the smaller acoustic window of the spleen compared with the liver. It is important to remember that the left kidney is located more cephalad than the right kidney. Examination of the splenorenal space is also obtained with caudad/cephalad and anterior/posterior sweeping motions of the probe between the rib interspaces. Fluid in this potential space also appears as a black stripe, but can be more difficult to identify compared with Morison's pouch as fluid can track anteriorly between the spleen and the abdominal wall (Fig. 4). After the splenorenal space has been fully examined, the left kidney, spleen, and thorax should also be examined, understanding that identifying splenic injuries can be difficult.

The suprapubic space (rectouterine or rectovesicular space depending on the sex of the patient) is examined next. An initial transverse view of this potential space is performed with the probe placed a few

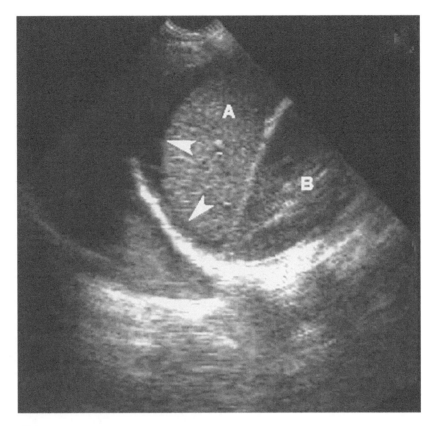

Figure 4
Fluid in the splenorenal space. Fluid is located superior and anterior to the spleen (A).

centimeters above the pubic symphysis angled caudad (Fig. 5). This location uses the bladder as an acoustic window and therefore should be performed prior to insertion of a foley. Although it is not practical in the trauma setting, instilling 250 cc of fluid into the bladder via the foley catheter increases the ability to detect intraperitoneal fluid. A caudad sweeping motion of the probe beam can identify free fluid posterior to the bladder (Fig. 6). Care must be taken not to confuse the prostate with free fluid, as the prostate can appear as an anechoic area if the beam is directed too far caudally. To add sensitivity to the suprapubic view, an additional longitudinal view of these structures can be performed.

The final view is the subxiphoid (subcostal) cardiac window, which is a focused, four-chambered look at the heart with the single goal of visualizing pericardial fluid (Fig. 7). This is unlike standard cardiac echocardiography, which is lengthy and incorporates numerous views of the myocardium and valvular structures for diagnosing cardiac pathology. With the probe in the subxiphoid location, the beam is directed to the patient's left shoulder providing a coronal section of

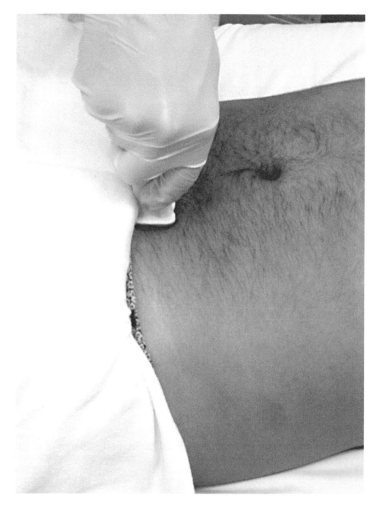

Figure 5
Suprapubic probe placement.

the heart and part of the liver. With sweeping views in the anterior/
posterior direction, the pericardium can be inspected for an anechoic
stripe surrounding the heart, in the space between the liver and the right
ventricle (Fig. 8).

BLUNT ABDOMINAL TRAUMA

Accuracy

The use of US to detect hemoperitoneum and abdominal injury has been
studied extensively in patients with blunt abdominal trauma. In recent
studies, the sensitivity and specificity range from 76% to 90% and 95%

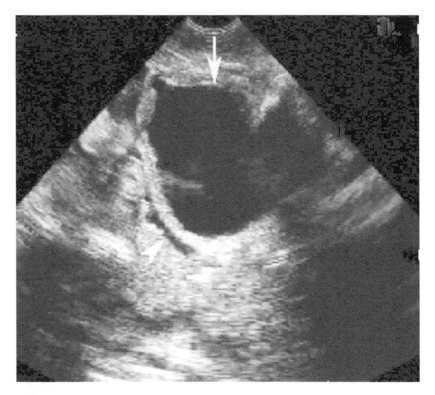

Figure 6
Fluid in the pelvis. The arrowhead points to fluid located posterior to the
bladder.

to 100%, respectively, for detecting hemoperitoneum as an indicator of
intraperitoneal injury (1,16–27). Surgeons, at various stages of training,
have been found to perform the examination with similar accuracy as
attending radiologists (28). In one study, as little as one hour of didactic
and one hour of practical training resulted in a sensitivity and specificity
of 75% and 96%, respectively, for detecting intraperitoneal fluid. The
accuracy increased with experience and practice (16).

As the primary goal of the trauma ultrasonography examination is
to detect hemoperitoneum, investigators have recently investigated the
rate of missed abdominal injuries in patients without hemoperitoneum,
evident during the FAST examination. Chiu et al. found that 29% of
52 patients with abdominal injury on CT had no evidence of hemoperitoneum on CT or ultrasonography. Four patients with splenic injury
required laparotomy while the remaining patients had nonoperative splenic and liver injuries. They also found that pain or tenderness, pulmonary
contusions, low rib fractures, hemothorax, pneumothorax, hematuria,
pelvic fractures, and thoracolumbar spine fractures were associated with
an increased risk of intraperitoneal injury without hemoperitoneum (11).
In a larger series of patients, Shanmuganathan et al. reported no evidence

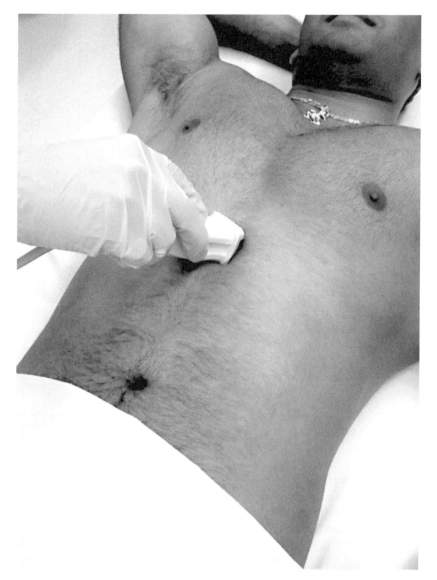

Figure 7
Subcoastal probe position.

of hemoperitoneum by CT in 34% of patients with abdominal visceral injuries. The most commonly missed injuries were splenic, hepatic, renal, mesenteric, and pancreatic injuries. Seventeen percent of the patients without hemoperitoneum required surgical or angiographic intervention for their injuries (29). In contrast, other studies suggest a sensitivity and specificity of 95% for detecting intraperitoneal injuries based on the findings of hemoperitoneum and actual organ parenchymal injury. In this study, 18% of these patients did not have hemoperitoneum. The

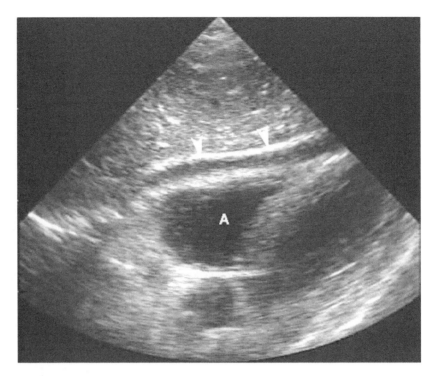

Figure 8
Pericardial effusion. The arrow heads point to pericardial fluid located in the
space between the liver (*above*) and the right ventricle (A).

sensitivities of ultrasonography for pancreatic and intestinal injuries were
only 71% and 35%, respectively (30). The main limitation of this study is
that the ultrasonographers attempted to identify specific organ parenchymal injuries. This technique requires more training and is fraught with
potential error as the sensitivity of ultrasonography for identifying specific organ injury is low (see below). The results from this experienced Japa-
nese US group have not been reproduced.

The incidence of a negative FAST examination in stable blunt
trauma patients with intraperitoneal injury can be quite high (8,31).
Poletti et al. (8) reported that 31% of hemodynamically stable patients
with organ injury did not have intraperitoneal free fluid, and 10% of these
patients required surgery or embolization. Based on these results, further
work-up for intraperitoneal injury is required despite a negative FAST
examination. The FAST examination should not be used to replace CT
scan in these patients.

The amount of intraperitoneal fluid detectable by US in trauma
patients has been studied in patients with ascites. In these patients, without cervical spine precautions and with optimal positioning, the least
amount of fluid detectible in Morison's pouch was 100 cc (32). Later
work in trauma patients found that the mean volume of fluid detected

by US was 619 cc. In this study, ultrasonographers performed examinations of Morison's pouch as DPL fluid was being infused to determine the amount of fluid that resulted in a positive examination. The authors reported that only 10% of ultrasonographers could detect < 400 mL while 97% could detect over 1 L (33). Simple physics dictates that patient position could alter the location of intraperitoneal fluid. One study looked at fluid visualization in trauma patients undergoing a DPL and found that when patients are placed in 5° of Trendelenburg, less intraperitoneal fluid was needed for ultrasonography visualization (400 cc vs. 700 cc) (34). This suggests that placing the patient in Trendelenberg may increase the sensitivity of the test. However, this position may decrease the sensitivity of ultrasonography for detecting hemothorax, and would be harmful in the head-injured patient with elevated intracranial pressure. A single supine FAST examination is still considered the optimal initial study.

Sensitivity of the FAST examination increases with the number of views obtained. The single Morison's pouch view had a sensitivity of 51% and specificity of 93% when used alone versus a sensitivity of 87% and specificity of 100% when multiple views were obtained. In this study, the multiple-view technique (six views) included the paracolic gutters (21). Ingeman reported sensitivities of 78%, 56%, and 58% for the Morison's pouch, suprapubic, and splenorenal views, respectively; the specificities were 97%, 100%, and 98%, respectively (16). If possible, multiple views should be obtained.

The accuracy of the FAST examination for identifying specific solid organ or hollow viscous injuries is low. The sensitivity of ultrasonography for splenic injury has been reported to be as low as 33% (17,35–37). Hepatic injuries are also difficult to identify with ultrasonography. Richards et al. reported a sensitivity of 67% when hemoperitoneum was used as the indicator of injury and 72% when hemoperitoneum and parenchymal abnormalities were used as criteria for a positive ultrasonography. Actual parenchymal injuries were detected in only 12% of patients. This study demonstrates the limitations of ultrasonography for identifying specific organ injuries and highlights that in the trauma setting, hemoperitoneum should be the primary finding used to indicate intraperitoneal injury (38). The same authors documented a sensitivity of 44% for the detection of isolated small bowel and mesenteric injuries based on the presence of free fluid. This compares with a sensitivity of 80% for CT scan (9). These injuries often are accompanied by minimal amounts of free intraperitoneal bleeding and therefore result in a negative FAST examination.

Clinical Algorithm

The management implications of the FAST results depend on the stability of the patient. A stable patient with systolic blood pressure > 90 mmHg should undergo ultrasonography followed by CT scan. Since physical examination findings alone are insensitive in predicting thoracic or abdominal injury, the determination of whether CT scan is indicated should be based on the mechanism of injury and the clinical presentation (17). Patients at risk for occult injuries such as small bowel injury or patients with pelvic or spine fractures should undergo CT. Some authors recommend that DPL or CT scan be performed in patients with a seat belt sign in the abdominal region, since these patients are at risk for small bowel and pancreatic injuries (26). It is also recommended that patients with persistent abdominal pain or tenderness undergo CT scanning since these patients are at increased risk for small bowel injury as well as for retroperitoneal hematomas (26,39). Rozycki et al. (40) prospectively studied patients with spine and pelvic fractures, and compared ultrasonography with CT results. The sensitivities of ultrasonography in these patients were significantly lower compared with other reported sensitivities. The results of this study are difficult to interpret, as many of the patients with false negative ultrasonography results actually had small amounts of pelvic fluid on CT scan and were managed nonoperatively. Injuries that were missed included renal, small bowel, diaphragm, and bladder injuries. The authors conclude that in patients with pelvic fractures, the rate of false negative FAST results is higher and thus CT is recommended.

The unstable blunt trauma patient presents a diagnostic challenge to the emergency physician and trauma surgeon. An immediate search for causes of hypotension is needed. Potential sources include intraperitoneal hemorrhage, chest injuries (hemothorax, pneumothorax, and cardiac tamponade), retroperitoneal hemorrhage associated with pelvic fractures, and neurogenic shock associated with spinal fractures. Less common causes include cardiac rupture. The accuracy and utility of ultrasonography in the unstable blunt trauma patient has been studied, although the numbers of patients in these studies are small. Lentz prospectively compared ultrasonography performed by a radiology resident, fellow, or technician to DPL results in 54 patients with systolic blood pressure ≤ 90 mmHg and found a sensitivity of 87% and specificity of 100%. In this study, there were two patients with false negative ultrasonography results, but only one of them required operative intervention. This patient had a splenic laceration with fluid loculated centrally in the abdomen due to adhesions from previous surgery (24). Thus, patients with previous abdominal surgery may require confirmatory CT or DPL, if the ultrasonography is negative. Wherrett et al. (5) had more promising results in 69 patients with hypotension. In their study, ultrasonography was performed at three sites (Morison's pouch, the pouch of Douglas, and the splenorenal space) and the results were compared with CT, DPL, and laparotomy results. The sensitivity of ultrasonography for predicting the need for an immediate laparotomy was 100%. However, one of the patients had a delayed laparotomy for evolving peritonitis from an isolated jejunal injury. In this study, none of the patients with a negative FAST examination required an immediate laparotomy for acute control of hemorrhage. The recommendations from this study are that ultrasonography can be used to exclude acute intraperitoneal hemorrhage as the cause of hypotension in blunt trauma patients. If the FAST is negative, then another source of hypotension should be suspected, such as retroperitoneal bleeding from pelvic fractures or neurogenic shock. The authors recommend that in patients with major pelvic trauma, a negative FAST should be followed by external fixation or angiography with embolization. The other option in the unstable patient with a negative initial FAST examination is to repeat the examination while the patient is still in the trauma room (10). This may increase the chances of detecting intraperitoneal bleeding. The conservative approach is to perform a DPL to confirm the negative result. In a more recent study, Rozycki et al. (40) documented 100% specificity and sensitivity in 30 hypotensive blunt trauma patients. This study compared ultrasonography to DPL, CT, and laparotomy findings for identifying intraperitoneal hemorrhage as the cause of hypotension. Because of the high sensitivity and specificity of ultrasonography, laparotomy should be performed when the ultrasonography is positive. Although the numbers of patients in these studies are small, these preliminary data suggest that a negative FAST examination may be used to exclude intraperitoneal bleeding as the cause of hypotension. The algorithm in Figure 9 summarizes the general approach to the blunt abdominal trauma patient.

The FAST examination may also be used as part of a clinical pathway for low mechanism blunt abdominal trauma patients to decrease the utilization of CT and hospital admission rate. Branney et al. (41) proposed a pathway utilizing an initial FAST examination followed by serial ultrasonography examinations and observation for 8 to 12 hours with serial physical examinations and hematocrits. Using this algorithm, they documented a decrease in CT scan use from 56% to 26% and a 38% decrease in the hospital admission rate. In the era of cost containment, as ultrasonography becomes more a part of standard practice in trauma centers, this may be a cost-saving approach to managing low mechanism trauma patients.

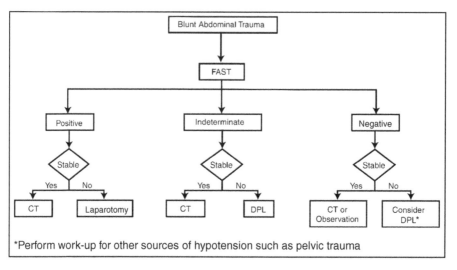

Figure 9
Blunt Abdominal Trauma Algorithm. *Source*: From Ref. 58.

DETECTION OF HEMOTHORAX

As previously discussed, an emergency physician or surgeon must be able to quickly diagnose major life-threatening injuries in an unstable trauma patient. Not only is the FAST examination accurate for the diagnosis of hemoperitoneum and hemopericardium, but it is also used in many trauma centers for the rapid detection of hemothorax (1,17,40,42). Surgeons with limited training in bedside ultrasonography can accurately and easily detect traumatic pleural effusions. In a prospective study of 360 patients (75% blunt and 25% penetrating trauma), 40 patients had traumatic effusions. Of these, 39 were detected by US and 37 were diagnosed by a standard supine portable radiograph. The supine chest X-ray was considered the gold standard in this study, although ultrasonography diagnosed three pleural effusions missed on the X-ray. The sensitivity (97.5%) and specificity (99.7%) for US were comparable to those of the supine chest X-ray (sensitivity 92.5%, specificity 99.7%). Notably, the results of the ultrasonography were obtained in an average of 1.3 minutes compared to 14 minutes for the chest X-ray (43). Another study also compared the FAST examination to chest radiography in 240 patients and found equivalent sensitivity (96.2%) and specificity (100%) for the detection of hemothorax. Two-thirds of the patients were victims of blunt trauma and 33% had penetrating chest injuries. In this study, chest CT, thoracostomy, or serial upright chest X-rays were used as the gold standard (44). Kimura and Otsuka (1) and Rothlin et al. (17) reported slightly lower accuracies for the detection of hemothorax (67% and 81% respectively). In contrast to these reports, Abboud and Kendall (45) recently published a series on blunt trauma patients with suspected hemothorax. Although the training of the physicians performing the examinations was comparable to that in previous studies, the authors reported missing 14 pleural effusions in 142 patients for an overall sensitivity of 12.5% and specificity of 98.4%. Further work is needed in this area to truly define the accuracy of bedside US for hemothorax in the setting of blunt trauma.

To diagnose a traumatic effusion, two additional views are added to the standard FAST examination, the right intercostal oblique and left intercostal oblique views. These views are easily obtained by first imaging Morison's pouch and the splenorenal space and shifting the probe superiorly to visualize the pleural cavity (Fig. 2). On US, fluid in the pleural space is seen as a hypoechoic space above the hyperechoic diaphragm (Fig. 10) (46).

Ultrasonography is not intended to replace the chest X-ray in the routine evaluation of the trauma patient. A chest radiograph is important for identifying mediastinal and bony injuries and a pneumothorax, and to check endotracheal, nasogastric, and chest tube placement. Bedside ultrasonography complements the supine chest X-ray by accurately and efficiently diagnosing a traumatic effusion.

Using ultrasonography in the trauma patient has several potential advantages. Bedside ultrasonography can be performed significantly

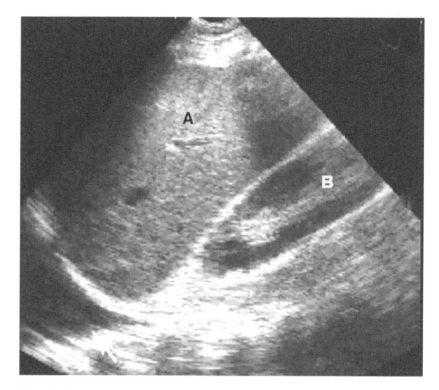

Figure 10
Hemothorax. The arrow points to hemothorax located superior to the hyperechoic diaphragm.

faster than a portable chest X-ray and can expedite the placement of a
thoracostomy tube prior to return of the initial chest X-ray results (43).
US can also accurately detect a smaller amount of pleural fluid than a
chest X-ray. US detects as little as 20 ml of fluid, compared to a minimum
of 175 mL on a supine chest radiograph (17,47). An upright chest X-ray
can detect 50 to 100 cc of pleural fluid. However, the majority of trauma
patients are immobilized on a long spine board and cannot be reposi-
tioned because of other potential injuries (48). US can also be used to distinguish pleural effusion from pulmonary contusion if the supine chest
X-ray is equivocal (44).

PENETRATING ABDOMINAL TRAUMA

The FAST examination clearly has a defined role in the initial assessment
of the blunt trauma patient (22,24,35,39,40,42,49). More recently, many
trauma centers have also started utilizing the FAST examination to
rapidly diagnose intraperitoneal hemorrhage in patients with penetrating
abdominal trauma (50). In these patients, US examination offers no additional benefit if the need for emergent surgery is apparent. The FAST

examination can be helpful in localizing the presence of significant hemorrhage in the patient with multiple wounds. This is especially important with wounds to the lower chest and epigastrium, as the FAST examination is used to guide interventions such as tube thoracostomy, pericardiocentesis, or laparotomy in the unstable patient (18).

As described above, ultrasonography depends on the presence of significant hemoperitoneum to detect intra-abdominal injuries. Herein lies the limitation of ultrasonography in the setting of penetrating abdominal trauma. Several authors have reported that the FAST examination will miss clinically significant intra-abdominal injuries such as to the bowel or diaphragm, if there is minimal hemorrhage (11,29,51).

In a recent study examining the routine use of the FAST examination in 72 patients with penetrating torso trauma, the sensitivity of the FAST examination for intra-abdominal injury was 67% and specificity was 92%. There were six patients with significant abdominal injuries that were missed by US. These included injuries to the liver, bowel, diaphragm (three patients), stomach, and omentum (50). Udobi et al. (52) prospectively evaluated the utility of ultrasonography in 75 patients with penetrating abdominal trauma. The FAST examination was positive for intraperitoneal hemorrhage in 21 patients and therapeutic laparotomy in 19. However, there were also 22 false negative FAST examinations (sensitivity 46%, specificity 94%). Thirteen of these patients had peritoneal blood at laparotomy and nine had injuries to the diaphragm or bowel requiring operative repair but with minimal associated hemorrhage. Both authors conclude that a positive FAST examination is a good predictor of injury and can be used to triage patients rapidly to the operating room. However, in the setting of penetrating trauma, a negative FAST examination should be followed by further diagnostic studies such as DPL, CT scan, or laparoscopy because of the potential for missed injuries.

PENETRATING CHEST TRAUMA

Timely detection of a pericardial effusion and cardiac tamponade in patients with penetrating chest trauma is one of the most important applications of emergency department ultrasonography (53). The classic physical examination findings of cardiac tamponade, such as muffled heart sounds, hypotension, and distended neck veins, are present in < 40% of confirmed cases, and may be difficult to assess in a busy trauma room (13). Many patients with significant cardiac injuries may not have overt signs until hemodynamic collapse occurs (14). Survival from a penetrating cardiac injury is dependent on the rapid diagnosis and management of a pericardial effusion and cardiac tamponade (54). Emergency echocardiography is a noninvasive and accurate method to quickly confirm the presence or absence of a pericardial effusion in these patients.

Several studies have demonstrated that ultrasonography performed by surgeons and emergency physicians is very sensitive for the detection of pericardial fluid. Rozycki et al. (55) examined 261 patients with penetrating chest injuries, and found a sensitivity of 100% and specificity of 96.9% for the detection of pericardial fluid. These authors recommend that bedside ultrasonography should be the initial diagnostic test in the evaluation of patients with penetrating chest trauma. It should be noted that the mean time from the ultrasonography to operative intervention was 12 minutes. Similarly, Mandavia et al. (53) demonstrated that emergency physicians correctly diagnosed a pericardial effusion with ultrasonography in 103 patients with a sensitivity of 96%, specificity of 98%, and an overall accuracy of 97.5%. The results in hemodynamically stable patients may be less impressive (sensitivity of 56% and specificity of 93%), though the authors noted that the high false negative rate in this study was found primarily in patients with a concurrent hemothorax. The sensitivity of ultrasonography for detecting occult cardiac injury was 100% in the group of patients without hemothorax (14).

In 1992, Plummer et al. (56) demonstrated that the use of emergency bedside echo improved the clinical outcome of 28 patients after penetrating cardiac trauma, as compared to a retrospective control group. Emergency echocardiography reduced the time from diagnosis to operative intervention from 42.4 ± 21.7 to 15.5 ± 11.4 minutes. Although both the echo and the control group had a probability of survival of 34% based on their injuries, the actual survival using echocardiography was 100% as compared to 57% in the control group.

Emergency bedside ultrasonography examination of the heart and pericardium is performed using a 2 to 3.5 MHz probe. The subxiphoid view is the standard position used for this examination and is ideal for the detection of pericardial fluid and cardiac tamponade (Fig. 7) (36). The parasternal long view can also be used if the subxiphoid view is technically limited by abdominal distention or other patient characteristics. The parasternal long axis view is obtained by placing the ultrasonography transducer to the left of the sternum in the third or fourth intercostal space, with the probe indicator directed toward the right shoulder. At this position, both ventricles are easily visualized. A pericardial effusion is seen as a dark or anechoic space between the heart and the pericardium. In the presence of a pericardial effusion, the echocardiographic signs of cardiac tamponade may also be seen. These include early diastolic collapse of the right ventricle and late diastolic collapse of the right atrium (13). Additionally, the inferior vena cava can be imaged in the subcostal region. Normally, the inferior vena cava collapses with a vigorous deep inspiration. In the setting of cardiac tamponade, the inferior vena cava will not collapse as the patient sniffs. This maneuver known as the Sniff Test is a useful indicator of elevated right heart pressure and may be technically easier to interpret than right ventricular diastolic collapse (36). The algorithm in Figure 11 summarizes the management of the penetrating chest trauma patient.

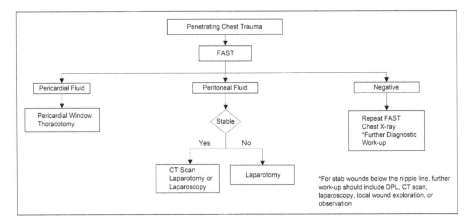

Figure 11
Penetrating chest trauma algorithm. *Source*: From Ref. 59.

SUMMARY

There are several pitfalls that must be avoided when performing the FAST examination. Multiple views should be obtained rather than just the Morison's pouch view, in order to increase the sensitivity of the test. In addition, serial examinations will increase the sensitivity and should be performed especially when there is a change in the clinical status of the patient. Finally, the limitations of the test should be considered. A negative test does not rule out the possibility of an intraperitoneal injury requiring an operation.

In summary, bedside ultrasonography has a critical role in the management of the blunt and penetrating trauma patient. In the blunt trauma patient, ultrasonography is used to triage patients to CT, the operating room, or the angiography suite. The FAST examination facilitates the performance of life-saving procedures such as tube thoracostomy. In the penetrating trauma patient, the primary use of ultrasonography is to detect cardiac injury in order to decrease the time to the operating room and definitive management. To achieve the desirable degree of accuracy and proficiency with the FAST examination, the American College of Emergency Physicians recommends a one-day training ultrasonography course with lectures and hands-on practical sessions with live models as an initial introductory course on the FAST examination. Experiential supervised training with the performance of 25 examinations should follow this (57). With this training and experience, emergency physicians and surgeons can use the FAST examination to significantly improve the care of the trauma patient.

REFERENCES

1. Kimura A, Otsuka T. Emergency center ultrasonography in the evaluation of hemoperitoneum: a prospective study. J Trauma 1991; 31(1):20–23.
2. Gruessner R, Mentges B, Duber C, Ruckert K, Rothmund M. Sonography versus peritoneal lavage in blunt abdominal trauma. J Trauma 1989; 29(2):242–244.
3. American College of Surgeons, Committee on Trauma. Advanced Trauma Life Support Instructor Course Manual. Chicago, Illinois, 1997.
4. Boulanger BR, Kearney PA, Brenneman FD, Tsuei B, Ochoa J. Utilization of FAST (Focused Assessment with Sonography for Trauma) in 1999: results of a survey of North American trauma centers. Am Surg 2000; 66(11):1049–1055.
5. Wherrett LJ, Boulanger BR, McLellan BA, Brenneman FD, Rizoli SB, Culhane J, Hamilton P. Hypotension after blunt abdominal trauma: the role of emergent abdominal sonography in surgical triage. J Trauma 1996; 41(5):815–820.
6. Boulanger BR, Brenneman FD, Kirkpatrick AW, McLellan BA, Nathens AB. The indeterminate abdominal sonogram in multisystem blunt trauma. J Trauma 1998; 45(1):52–56.
7. Henderson SO, Sung J, Mandavia D. Serial abdominal ultrasound in the setting of trauma. J Emerg Med 2000; 18(1):79–81.
8. Poletti PA, Kinkel K, Vermeulen B, Irmay F, Unger PF, Terrier F. Blunt abdominal trauma: should US be used to detect both free fluid and organ injuries? Radiology 2003; 227(1):95–103.
9. Richards JR, McGahan JP, Simpson JL, Tabar P. Bowel and mesenteric injury: evaluation with emergency abdominal US. Radiology 1999; 211(2):399–403.
10. Boulanger BR, McLellan BA, Brenneman FD, Wherrett L, Rizoli SB, Culhane J, Hamilton P. Emergent abdominal sonography as a screening test in a new diagnostic algorithm for blunt trauma. J Trauma 1996; 40(6):867–874.
11. Chiu WC, Cushing BM, Rodriguez A, Ho SM, Mirvis SE, Shanmuganathan K, Stein M. Abdominal injuries without hemoperitoneum: a potential limitation of focused abdominal sonography for trauma (FAST). J Trauma 1997; 42(4):617–623 [discussion 623–625].
12. Plummer D. The sensitivity, specificity, and accuracy of ED echocardiography. Acad Emerg Med 1995; 2:339.
13. Chan D. Echocardiography in thoracic trauma. Emerg Med Clin North Am 1998; 16(1):191–207.
14. Meyer DM, Jessen ME, Grayburn PA. Use of echocardiography to detect occult cardiac injury after penetrating thoracic trauma: a prospective study. J Trauma 1995; 39(5):902–907 [discussion 907–909].
15. Meyers MA. The spread and localization of acute intraperitoneal effusions. Radiology 1970; 95(3):547–554.
16. Ingeman JE, Plewa MC, Okasinski RE, King RW, Knotts FB. Emergency physician use of ultrasonography in blunt abdominal trauma. Acad Emerg Med 1996; 3(10):931–937.
17. Rothlin MA, Naf R, Amgwerd M, Candinas D, Frick T, Trentz O. Ultrasound in blunt abdominal and thoracic trauma. J Trauma 1993; 34(4):488–495.
18. Rozycki GS, Ochsner MG, Schmidt JA, Frankel HL, Davis TP, Wang D, Champion HR. A prospective study of surgeon-performed ultrasound as the primary adjuvant modality for injured patient assessment. J Trauma 1995; 39(3):492–498; [discussion 498–500].
19. Rozycki GS, Ochsner MG, Jaffin JH, Champion HR. Prospective evaluation of surgeons' use of ultrasound in the evaluation of trauma patients. J Trauma 1993; 34(4):516–526; [discussion 526–527].

20. Ma OJ, Mateer JR, Ogata M, Kefer MP, Wittmann D, Aprahamian C. Prospective analysis of a rapid trauma ultrasound examination performed by emergency physicians. J Trauma 1995; 38(6):879–885.

21. Ma OJ, Kefer MP, Mateer JR, Thoma B. Evaluation of hemoperitoneum using a single-vs multiple-view ultrasonographic examination. Acad Emerg Med 1995; 2(7):581–586.

22. Hoffmann R, Nerlich M, Muggia-Sullam M, Pohlemann T, Wippermann B, Regel G, Tscherne H. Blunt abdominal trauma in cases of multiple trauma evaluated by ultrasonography: a prospective analysis of 291 patients. J Trauma 1992; 32(4):452–458.

23. Tso P, Rodriguez A, Cooper C, Militello P, Mirvis S, Badellino MM, Boulanger BR, Foss FA Jr, Hinson DM, Mighty HE, et al. Sonography in blunt abdominal trauma: a preliminary progress report. J Trauma 1992; 33(1):39–43; [discussion 43–44].

24. Lentz KA, McKenney MG, Nunez DB Jr, Martin L. Evaluating blunt abdominal trauma: role for ultrasonography. J Ultrasound Med 1996; 15(6):447–451.

25. McElveen TS, Collin GR. The role of ultrasonography in blunt abdominal trauma: a prospective study. Am Surg 1997; 63(2):184–188.

26. Rozycki GS, Ochsner MG, Feliciano DV, Thomas B, Boulanger BR, Davis FE, Falcone RE, Schmidt JA. Early detection of hemoperitoneum by ultrasound examination of the right -upper quadrant: a multicenter study. J Trauma 1998; 45(5):878–883.

27. Bode PJ, Edwards MJ, Kruit MC, van Vugt AB. Sonography in a clinical algorithm for early evaluation of 1671 patients with blunt abdominal trauma. Am J Roentgenol 1999; 172(4):905–911.

28. McKenney MG, McKenney KL, Compton RP, Namias N, Fernandez L, Levi D, Arrillaga A, Lynn M, Martin L. Can surgeons evaluate emergency ultrasound scans for blunt abdominal trauma? J Trauma 1998; 44(4):649–653.

29. Shanmuganathan K, Mirvis SE, Sherbourne CD, Chiu WC, Rodriguez A. Hemoperitoneum as the sole indicator of abdominal visceral injuries: a potential limitation of screening abdominal US for trauma. Radiology 1999; 212(2):423–430.

30. Yoshii H, Sato M, Yamamoto S, Motegi M, Okusawa S, Kitano M, Nagashima A, Doi M, Takuma K, Kato K, Aikawa N. Usefulness and limitations of ultrasonography in the initial evaluation of blunt abdominal trauma. J Trauma 1998; 45(1):45–50; [discussion 50—51].

31. Miller MT, Pasquale MD, Bromberg WJ, Wasser TE, Cox J. Not so FAST. J Trauma 2003; 54(1):52–59; [discussion 59–60].

32. Goldberg BB, Clearfield HR, Goodman GA, Morales JO. Ultrasonic determination of ascites. Arch Intern Med 1973; 131(2):217–220.

33. Branney SW, Wolfe RE, Moore EE, Albert NP, Heining M, Mestek M, Eule J. Quantitative sensitivity of ultrasound in detecting free intraperitoneal fluid. J Trauma 1995; 39(2):375–380.

34. Abrams BJ, Sukumvanich P, Seibel R, Moscati R, Jehle D. Ultrasound for the detection of intraperitoneal fluid: the role of Trendelenburg positioning. Am J Emerg Med 1999; 17(2):117–120.

35. Bennett MK, Jehle D. Ultrasonography in blunt abdominal trauma. Emerg Med Clin North Am 1997; 15(4):763–787.

36. Rosen CL, Branney SW, Wolfe RE. Emergency ultrasound. In: Rosen P, Barkin R, Danzl D, Hockberger RS, Ling LJ, Markovchick V, Marx JA, Newton E, Walls RM, eds. Emergency Medicine Concepts and Clinical Practice. 4th ed. St. Louis: Mosby, 1998:188–196.

37. Nordenholz KE, Rubin MA, Gularte GG, Liang HK. Ultrasound in the evaluation and management of blunt abdominal trauma. Ann Emerg Med 1997; 29(3):357–366.

38. Richards JR, McGahan JP, Pali MJ, Bohnen PA. Sonographic detection of blunt hepatic trauma: hemoperitoneum and parenchymal patterns of injury. J Trauma 1999; 47(6):1092–1097.

39. Glaser K, Tschmelitsch J, Klingler P, Wetscher G, Bodner E. Ultrasonography in the management of blunt abdominal and thoracic trauma. Arch Surg 1994; 129(7):743–747.

40. Rozycki GS, Ballard RB, Feliciano DV, Schmidt JA, Pennington SD. Surgeon-performed ultrasound for the assessment of truncal injuries: lessons learned from 1540 patients. Ann Surg 1998; 228(4):557–567.

41. Branney SW, Moore EE, Cantrill SV, Burch JM, Terry SJ. Ultrasound -based key clinical pathway reduces the use of hospital resources for the evaluation of blunt abdominal trauma. J Trauma 1997; 42(6):1086–1090.

42. Rozycki GS, Newman PG. Surgeon-performed ultrasound for the assessment of abdominal injuries. Adv Surg 1999; 33:243–259.

43. Sisley AC, Rozycki GS, Ballard RB, Namias N, Salomone JP, Feliciano DV. Rapid detection of traumatic effusion using surgeon-performed ultrasonography. J Trauma 1998; 44(2):291–296; [discussion 296–297].

44. Ma OJ, Mateer JR. Trauma ultrasound examination versus chest radiography in the detection of hemothorax. Ann Emerg Med 1997; 29(3):312–315; [discussion 315–316].

45. Abboud P, Kendall, J. Emergency department ultrasound for hemothorax after blunt traumatic injury. J Emerg Med 2003; 25(2):181–184.

46. Ma OJ, Mateer J. Trauma. In: Ma OJ, Mateer J, eds. Emergency Ultrasound. New York: McGraw-Hill, 2003:67–88.

47. Juhl J. Diseases of the pleura, mediastinum, and diaphragm. In: Juhl JH, Crummy AB, ed. Essentials of Radiologic Imaging. 6th ed. Philadelphia: JB Lippincott, 1993:1026.

48. Rubens M. The pleura:collapse and consolidation. In: Sutton D, ed. A Textbook of Radiology Imaging. Edinburgh: Churchill Livingstone, 1987:393.

49. Goletti O, Ghiselli, G, Lippolis, PV, Chiarugi, M, Braccini, G, Macaluso, C, Cavina, E. The role of ultrasonography in blunt abdominal trauma: results in 250 consecutive cases. J Trauma 1994; 36(2):178–181.

50. Boulanger BR, Kearney PA, Tsuei B, Ochoa JB. The routine use of sonography in penetrating torso injury is beneficial. J Trauma 2001; 51(2):320–325.

51. Sherbourne CD. Visceral injuries without peritoneum: a limitation of screening abdominal ultrasonography for trauma. Emerg Radiol 1997:349–354.

52. Udobi KF, Rodriguez A, Chiu WC, Scalea TM. Role of ultrasonography in penetrating abdominal trauma: a prospective clinical study. J Trauma 2001; 50(3):475–479.

53. Mandavia DP, Hoffner RJ, Mahaney K, Henderson SO. Bedside echocardiography by emergency physicians. Ann Emerg Med 2001; 38(4):377–382.

54. Rohman M, Ivatury RR, Steichen FM, Gaudino J, Nallathambi MN, Khan M, Stahl WM. Emergency room thoracotomy for penetrating cardiac injuries. J Trauma 1983; 23(7):570–576.

55. Rozycki GS, Feliciano DV, Ochsner MG, Knudson MM, Hoyt DB, Davis F, Hammerman D, Figueredo V, Harviel JD, Han DC, Schmidt JA. The role of ultrasound in patients with possible penetrating cardiac wounds: a prospective multicenter study. J Trauma 1999; 46(4):543–551; [discussion 51–2].

56. Plummer D, Brunette D, Asinger R, Ruiz E. Emergency department echocardiography improves outcome in penetrating cardiac injury. Ann Emerg Med 1992; 21(6):709–712.

57. ACEP Emergency Ultrasound Guidelines-2001. http://www.acep.org, 2001.

58. Rosen CL, Promes SB. Use of ultrasound in emergency medicine. Clinical Bulletin, Second Quarter 2003, Vol. VII, No. 2.

59. Tayal VS, Moore CL, Rose GA. Cardiar. In: Ma OJ, Mateer J, eds. Emergency Ultrasound. New York: McGraw-Hill, 2003:89–127.

7

Emergent Pelvic Ultrasound

Chris Moore
Department of Surgery, Section of Emergency Medicine, Yale University School of Medicine, New Haven, Connecticut, U.S.A.

Sonography is a key tool in the evaluation of the female patient with acute pelvic pain or vaginal bleeding. In early pregnancy, sonography can confirm the presence of intrauterine pregnancy (IUP), making an ectopic or extrauterine gestation (EUG) much less likely. In the non-pregnant female, ultrasound (US) may detect ovarian torsion or tubo-ovarian abscess. Ovarian cysts, while typically benign, may be easily identified by US and may help identify a cause for pelvic pain. US of the pelvis is particularly sensitive for free fluid which may indicate abdominal or pelvic hemorrhage.

The US can often be easily performed at the bedside by the clinician and has been shown to expedite care (1–4). This chapter will focus on basic techniques for performing both transabdominal and transvaginal pelvic US. Particular attention will be paid to the topic of ectopic pregnancy. Detection of common adnexal pathology will be briefly discussed, although comprehensive adnexal US is outside the scope of this text.

APPROACH TO PELVIC ULTRASOUND

When considering pelvic US, attention is often focused on the transvaginal approach. While this approach provides superior images, it may not always be the best first approach. Transvaginal sonography is more invasive and requires attention to chaperoning and infection control issues. In addition, sonographic orientation for this approach may be more difficult, especially for less experienced sonographers. Transabdominal US may be adequate for certain situations, and should generally be performed prior to transvaginal imaging.

Pelvic Anatomy and Ultrasound

The bladder is anterior and forms a key landmark for pelvic imaging. In the transabdominal approach, a full bladder provides an acoustic "window" that allows visualization of the rest of the pelvis. However, a full bladder is an impediment to transvaginal ultrasound (TVUS). A full bladder interferes with the transvaginal image and also physically pushes the uterus more posteriorly, making imaging more difficult.

The vaginal canal runs posterior and inferior to the bladder, terminating at the cervix. On transabdominal imaging, the "vaginal stripe," a hyperechoic (bright) line, may be seen that indicates the border (potential space) between the anterior and posterior vaginal walls. With transvaginal imaging, the vaginal stripe is not visualized as the transducer occupies this space. The uterus begins with the cervix, posterior to the bladder, and when in the typical anteverted position, bends anteriorly over the bladder. Approximately 10% of females have a retroverted uterus, which can make transabdominal imaging nearly impossible and transvaginal imaging confusing.

The ovaries are oblong and typically situated anterior and medial to the internal iliac vessels. Ovaries are often not visualized on transabdominal sonography, but may be seen if they are enlarged or contain cysts.

There are two potential spaces for fluid in the pelvis. The recto-uterine space, or Pouch of Douglas, is the most dependent, and often contains a small amount of nonpathologic fluid. The uterovesicular space is anterior to the uterus. It takes a large amount of fluid in the pelvis for the fluid to be found here. Fluid from the pelvis may flow into the abdominal cavity, and if a large amount is present, may be detected by the US in the hepatorenal space (Morrison's pouch).

Transabdominal Approach and Findings

Ideally the bladder is full when performing a transabdominal pelvic ultrasound, providing an acoustic window and minimizing interference from bowel gas, although this may not be essential (especially later in pregnancy). Typically a curvilinear probe in the 2.5 to 5 MHz frequency range is used. Beginning with a transverse view, the US probe is placed just cephalad to the symphysis pubis with the probe indicator directed to the patient's right side. The probe is angled inferiorly, so that the bladder is visualized, with the vaginal stripe and cervix posterior to the bladder. This transverse US image is oriented similarly to a cross-sectional computed tomography (CT) scan, with structures on the patient's right seen on the left side of the screen as seen by the sonographer (Fig. 1). The pelvis should be scanned completely in the transverse plane by sweeping the angle of the probe from the top of the uterus to the cervix.

After completing a transverse scan of the uterus, the probe should be rotated clockwise so that the probe indicator is towards the patient's head, providing a longitudinal (or sagittal) view. In this view, the bladder is seen anteriorly and inferiorly, with the vaginal stripe posterior (Fig. 2).

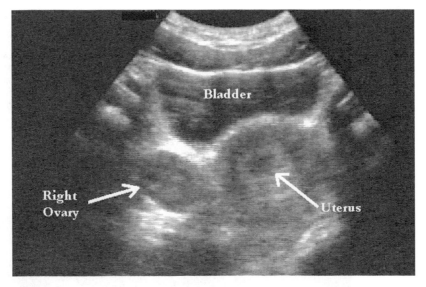

Figure 1
Transverse transabdominal image. The probe is just above the symphysis pubis with the indicator to the patient's right. The bladder is seen anteriorly with the uterus behind the bladder. Right-sided structures are on the left of the screen as it is viewed.

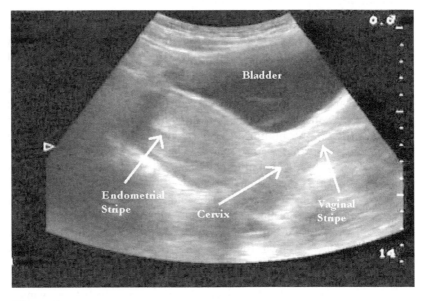

Figure 2
Sagittal (longitudinal) transabdominal image. The indicator is to the patient's head. The vaginal stripe is seen behind the bladder, leading to the cervix. The anteverted uterus is over the bladder.

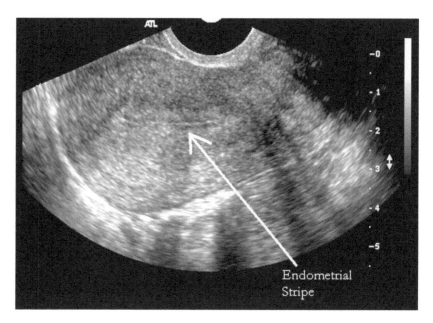

Endometrial
Stripe

Figure 3
Sagittal transvaginal image. The bladder is empty and is not seen. The uterine
fundus is superior, and the endometrial stripe is clearly seen.

Transvaginal Approach and Findings

It is essential that the patient empties her bladder before transvaginal images are taken. A small footprint, higher frequency (typically
5–9 MHz) intracavitary probe with cover or condom is used. It is important that gel be both between the cover and transducer as well as on
the outside of the cover. The probe should be held with the thumb placed
on an indicator that corresponds to the left side of the screen as you face
it. Transducer orientation should be confirmed prior to insertion of the
probe. Orientation in transvaginal scanning is more challenging due to
the fact that the probe is internal.

In the longitudinal plane, the indicator (thumb) should be up
(towards the ceiling). Looking at the screen in this orientation, the left
side of the screen is anterior and the right side is posterior. As the probe
is inserted in the vaginal vault, the cervix should come into view. Typically, the end of the probe will be on the cervix or in one of the fornices.
In most women, the uterus is anteverted and thus the cervix will curve
towards the uterine fundus from right to left on the screen (Fig. 3). If
the bladder is visualized at all, it will be anterior, on the left side of the
screen near the transducer. In approximately 10% of women the uterus
is retroverted, and will thus bend away from the bladder, towards the
right side of the screen as it is viewed (Fig. 4). Posterior to the cervix is
the Pouch of Douglas (rectouterine pouch), the most dependent area of
the pelvis and the area where pelvic fluid will collect if present (Fig. 5).

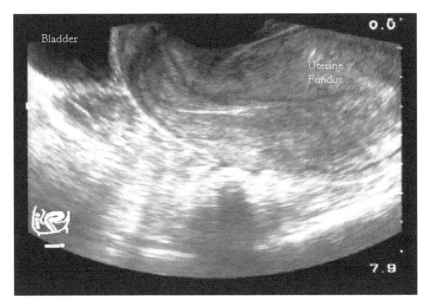

Figure 4
Retroverted uterus. The bladder is seen in the correct place, but the uterus is bending posteriorly.

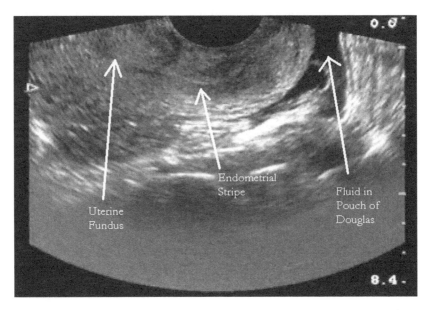

Figure 5
Sagittal transvaginal image, moderate free fluid in the rectouterine pouch (Pouch of Douglas).

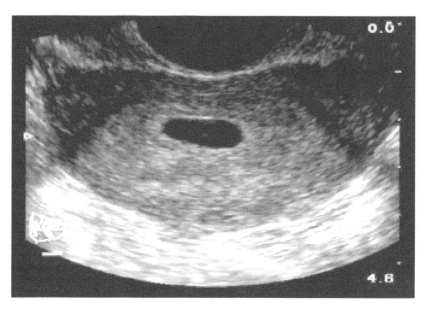

Figure 6
Coronal transvaginal image, with gestational sac. This is analogous to a transverse transabdominal image, although the bladder is empty and not seen.

The longitudinal view should include the uterus to the top of the fundus and then be swept from left to right to image the entire uterus.

Following longitudinal imaging, the probe should be rotated counterclockwise so that the examiner's thumb is to the patient's right. This provides a transverse or coronal image. In this orientation the left side of the screen is the patient's right, similar to a CT scan or transabdominal image (Fig. 6). Again the probe should be swept, this time from top to bottom in order to image the uterus from fundus to cervix.

ULTRASOUND IN EARLY PREGNANCY

Although the patient with a first trimester pregnancy presenting to the emergency department (ED) with pelvic pain or bleeding may have any number of pathologic conditions, by far the most frequent indication for pelvic US is to diagnose or exclude ectopic pregnancy or EUG. We will review the pathophysiology of EUG, the significance of the β-hCG level, and US findings in early pregnancy.

Ectopic Pregnancy

Ectopic pregnancy, also known as EUG, is the top cause of maternal mortality in the first trimester and has increased in incidence over the last several decades in the United States (5). EUG is estimated to occur in approximately 2% of pregnancies overall, but as many as 8% of women presenting to the ED with complaints related to early pregnancy may harbor an EUG (6–9).

While various algorithms incorporating clinical and laboratory variables have been proposed, US remains the test of choice in the evaluation of the pregnant patient who presents with abdominal pain or vaginal bleeding.

Risk factors for ectopic pregnancy include: prior pelvic surgery, previous EUG, intrauterine device use, previous genital infections, and smoking (6). However, nearly half of ectopic pregnancies occur in patients with no risk factors. The most common presentations of EUG include abdominal pain (present in 97% of patients) and vaginal bleeding (present in 87% of patients); but history and physical examination alone are neither sensitive nor specific for the diagnosis (8). Prior to the more widespread availability of ED ultrasound, it was estimated that as many as 40% of EUGs were missed on initial presentation (10). With liberal US use, sensitivity and specificity should exceed 90% (11).

Occasionally, US may definitively detect an EUG. However, more typically, the utility of US is in confirmation of an IUP, which makes simultaneous EUG (i.e., heterotopic pregnancy) unlikely. The exact incidence of heterotopic pregnancy is unknown, and estimates have ranged from 1/2600 to 1/30,000 pregnancies (12,13). Incidence increases with age and multiparity. The visualization of an IUP in the presence of fertility agents cannot be considered adequate to rule out ectopic gestation. The symptomatic patient with risk factors for heterotopic pregnancy should undergo the most thorough imaging available, in consultation with the obstetrician (14).

Even in the absence of fertility agents, a patient with an IUP and no ectopic pregnancy visualized by US still may harbor a heterotopic pregnancy. All patients presenting for rule-out ectopic pregnancy should be given thorough discharge instructions with follow-up unsured. Verification of IUP, though reassuring, does not completely eliminate the possibility of EUG (1). It is also possible for a patient to harbor more than one ectopic pregnancy simultaneously (15).

If an EUG is discovered or suspected, US may play a role in determining whether to pursue medical or surgical management. Methotrexate treatment for ectopic pregnancies may be appropriate with a β-hCG $< 15,000\,\text{mIU/mL}$, adnexal mass $< 3.5\,\text{cm}$, and minimal free pelvic fluid (7). Lower β-hCGs ($< 10,000\,\text{mIU/mL}$) are the strongest predictor of success with this treatment (16). EUGs that demonstrate cardiac activity or rupture with significant bleeding should be treated surgically.

β-hCG

While this chapter is primarily about US in pregnancy, understanding the relationship between β-hCG level and US findings is important. β-hCG is a hormone secreted by the placenta that rises predictably, nearly doubling every 48 hours in early pregnancy. Pregnancy is often first detected using a qualitative urine β-hCG test, with serum β-hCG measured when the quantitative level is desired. Although urine pregnancy tests used by hospitals and those available over-the-counter differ in sensitivity, most are quite sensitive and the best detect levels as low as 1 mIU/mL (17,18). However, a negative urine pregnancy test does not completely exclude pregnancy.

Studies correlating β-hCG with US examinations have resulted in the concept of the "discriminatory zone": the β-hCG level at which an IUP should be visualized by US with near 100% sensitivity (19). This level is generally agreed to be between 1000 and 2000 mIU/mL, and is frequently cited to be 1500 mIU/mL, although it may vary between different institutions (7,9,19–21). The discriminatory zone for trans-abdominal sonography is less well defined, but has been suggested to be between 4000 and 6500 mIU/mL (22,23).

There is no minimum β-hCG level at which an EUG rupture may occur (9). The risk of rupture peaks when the β-hCG approaches 1000 mIU/mL, but in one series of 131 patients with ruptured EUG, it was found that 57% ruptured at a level below 1000 mIU/mL, with 8% below 300 mIU/mL, and 2% below 100 mIU/mL (24,25). Although infrequent, an EUG rupture can occur and present dramatically even when the urine β-hCG is negative (26).

If an EUG is suspected, it is reasonable to obtain an ultrasound regardless of β-hCG level. Awaiting results of the β-hCG prior to performance of the ultrasound usually only delays patient care (7,27). Even with a β-hCG below 500 mIU/mL, US may still identify a significant percentage of EUGs (24). While some authors have recommended withholding US in stable patients who have a β-hCG of < 1500 mIU/mL (28), the largest published protocol, using this algorithm, recommended that over a third of patients with ectopics (69 out of 167) be discharged without having US performed (9,29). While US is certainly less sensitive with a lower β-hCG, it is likely that more than a third of these ectopics could have been identified prior to discharge, and others could have had an IUP confirmed.

The patient who presents with a β-hCG below the discriminatory zone, and an indeterminate US could represent any of three possibilities: EUG, early IUP, or spontaneous abortion. Consideration of the clinical picture and consultation with the obstetricians/gynecologists to assure continuity of care are important. In the stable patient, rechecking the β-hCG 48 hours later in an outpatient setting may be indicated (7). The β-hCG in patient with a normal IUP will double during this time period. A decline in β-hCG of > 50% indicates a low likelihood of EUG and most likely represents a spontaneous abortion. A slowly increasing β-hCG (< 66%), especially in the setting of an empty uterus by US, is highly indicative of an EUG (odds ratio 24.7) (21,30).

If β-hCG is above the discriminatory zone and no IUP is visualized, many obstetricians may opt to perform a dilatation and curettage

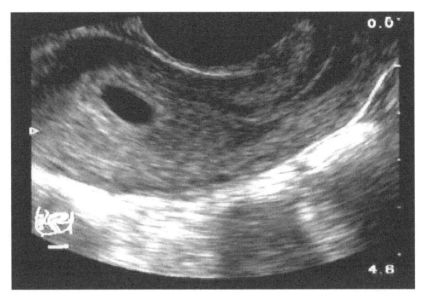

Figure 7
Sagittal transvaginal image with a gestational sac seen. There is a double decidual sac sign seen.

(D&C). Presence of chorionic villi provides evidence that this pregnancy represents a spontaneous abortion, while an absence indicates likely EUG. Some recommend that all women undergo a D&C prior to initiation of methotrexate therapy for EUG, although this is debatable (19,31).

Ultrasound Findings in Early Pregnancy

US in early pregnancy typically allows the classification of the patient into one of three categories: IUP, visualized EUG, or no definitive intrauterine pregnancy (NDIUP). As mentioned above, a visualized IUP makes an EUG unlikely. Assessment of fluid in the pelvis should also be performed.

Gestational Sac

The gestational sac is a circular, anechoic intrauterine area that should be visualized by approximately 4 to 5 weeks transvaginally (β-hCG of 1000–2000 mIU/mL) or five to six weeks transabdominally. It should be surrounded by a slightly thickened, echogenic rim that represents the border of the chorionic cavity (Fig. 7). Absence of this characteristic border may indicate a psuedogestational sac, which can develop with EUG (32). Although a true gestational sac is indicative of IUP, the differentiation between a true- and a pseudogestational sac is sometimes difficult. It is recommended that the presence of a gestational sac alone

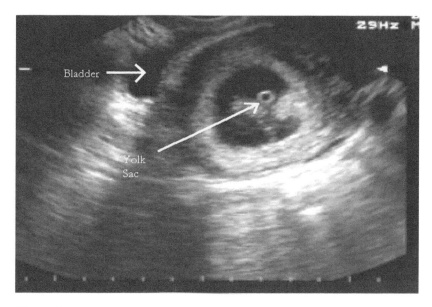

Figure 8
Coronal transvaginal image, intrauterine pregnancy with yolk sac (*long arrow*) and fetal pole.

should not be considered definitive evidence of IUP, especially when a novice sonographer is involved (33).

Double Decidual Sac Sign

The "double sac" sign was first described by Bradley et al. in 1982 as a US finding to diagnose early IUP in the absence of embryonic findings (34). While the hormones involved in EUG can cause thickening of the endometrial lining ("decidual cast"), a true IUP should involve the development of both the decidua parietalis and the deciduas capsularis, creating a pattern of concentric rings in the endometrial cavity. While it is still considered by many to be the earliest ultrasonographic sign of IUP, it is neither 100% sensitive nor specific for IUP and should be interpreted with caution (35).

Yolk Sac

The yolk sac is the first true embryonic landmark, appearing by about five weeks with TVUS. The yolk sac has a characteristic appearance of an echogenic ring approximately 5 mm in diameter within the gestational sac (Fig. 8). In a first trimester pregnancy with the estimated gestational age between 5 and 10 weeks, the upper limit for a normal developing yolk sac is 5.6 mm (36). In a normal IUP, a yolk sac should be visualized by the time the gestational sac reaches 8 to 10 mm. Visualization of a yolk sac is the first definitive evidence of IUP (33).

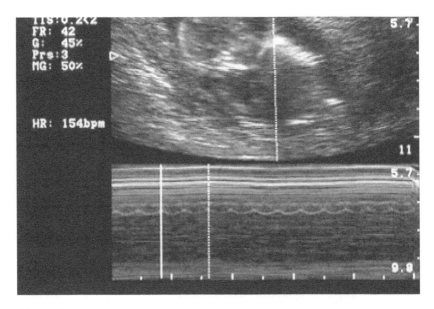

Figure 9
Fetal heart rate measured. The upper image is a two-dimensional image.
The dotted line across the upper image is the line displayed over time
in the lower m-mode image. The heart rate is measured over two cardiac
cycles.

Fetal Pole, Heart Tones

A fetal pole should be visualized by the time the gestational sac reaches
16 mm. Once the fetal pole has reached 5 mm, a cardiac flicker should
be visualized by TVUS (37). Fetal heart rate increases with increasing
size, and fetal bradycardia may represent impending fetal loss. A normal
fetus of less than 5 mm, 5 to 9 mm, and 10 to 15 mm should have a heart
rate of at least 100, 110, and 120 beats per minute, respectively (36). The
m-mode method of measuring fetal heart rate is described below and is
shown in Figure 9.

Abnormal Pregnancy

As the gestational sac enlarges, the yolk sac should be visualized,
followed by the fetal pole with cardiac activity. With TVUS, a gestational sac over 10 mm with no yolk sac or a gestational sac over
16 mm with no fetal pole can be considered abnormal. This is typically
called an anembryonic gestation or blighted ovum (37).

Subchorionic Hemorrhage

Subchorionic hemorrhage, also known as "implantation bleed," is
bleeding between the placental margin and uterine wall, typically

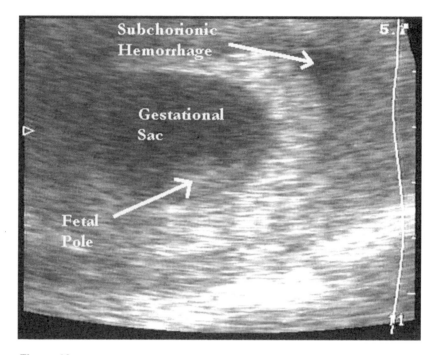

Figure 10
Subchorionic hemorrhage. The crescentic hemorrhage is seen just beneath the gestational sac.

appearing as a hypoechoic crescent in this area (Fig. 10) (36). Subchorionic hemorrhage is the most frequent cause of first trimester vaginal bleeding (37). The overall rate of miscarriage with subchorionic hemorrhage is approximately 9%, increasing with maternal age and size of the hematoma (38). Subchorionic hemorrhage also predisposes the patient to subsequent preterm labor and placental abruption, although it may spontaneously resolve without sequelae (39).

Extrauterine Gestation—Ectopic Pregnancy

While EUG may be suggested by a US that demonstrates an empty uterus with the presence of free pelvic fluid, more definitive evidence is provided by direct visualization of the ectopic pregnancy (Fig. 11). The most frequent sonographic evidence of ectopic pregnancy is a complex adnexal mass in the absence of an IUP. Occasionally, a true EUG with yolk sac and/or fetal pole with cardiac flicker may be seen. A live fetus may be seen in approximately one quarter of EUGs (36), if the procedure is performed by a skilled sonographer. More commonly, a "tubal ring" is visualized in the adnexa, indicating an embryo developing in a thickening fallopian tube. Most EUGs are clearly seen outside of the uterus, but in certain types of ectopic pregnancies may be misinterpreted as an IUP

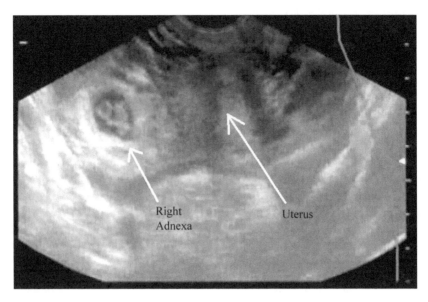

Figure 11
Ectopic pregnancy with tubal ring and yolk sac. This is seen in the right adnexa, apart from the uterus.

(10,41,42). The myometrial walls of the uterus come together at a junction known as the cornual point, which marks the beginning of the interstitial portion of the fallopian tube. Pregnancies may be found at any portion of this continuum: subcornual, cornual (including angular), and interstitial (41–45).

While true interstitial pregnancies represent < 1% of ectopic gestations, if rupture occurs it can be catastrophic due to the massive bleeding that may occur if this vascular portion of the fallopian tube at the edge of the uterus is disrupted (46,47).

It is imperative that the sonographer sees myometrium surrounding the entire gestation sac and that the myometrial rim be at least 8 mm thick to help rule out the cornual ectopic pregnancy.

Gestational Trophoblastic Disorder

Gestational trophoblastic disorders, also known as molar pregnancies, may be partial, complete, or invasive (choriocarcinoma). The most common type, a complete mole, represents a pregnancy where all embryonic DNA is paternal in origin. Sonographically, the typical appearance of a complete mole is that of an enlarged uterus with multiple small cystic areas, often referred to as a "cluster of grapes." Transabdominal sonography, with its wider field of view, may provide for an easier view of this disorder. Patients with molar pregnancies, typically associated with extremely high β-hCG levels, should undergo D&C and monitoring to watch for progression to invasive forms (48).

Retained Products of Conception

When patients present with significant symptoms after miscarriage, delivery, or operative intervention, there may be a concern regarding retained products of conception. US often determines whether expectant management, medical management, or operative intervention is required (49,50). Diagnosis of retained products should be considered when significant debris remain in the uterus, with an endometrial stripe over 8 mm, although some consider this overly conservative (51). Color Doppler may also be useful, with retained products demonstrating flow in the uterine wall.

ULTRASOUND IN LATER PREGNANCY

While US is used extensively in obstetrics and gynecology during later pregnancy, emergent indications for US in later pregnancy are more limited. They include the assessment of conditions that may be present in the nonpregnant patient, assessment of fetal age, viability, and evaluation for placental pathology.

Fetal Heart Rate

While a simple fetal Doppler instrument may serve the purpose of detecting fetal heart tones, US is also an excellent tool for visualizing fetal cardiac activity. Typically the heart is visualized in a 2-D image, and then m-mode is applied to measure it. M-mode ("motion" mode) involves the placement of a 1-D line over the 2-D image. This line is then displayed over time, with time forming the *x*-axis. This provides a still image that represents the beating heart. Heart rate is typically measured by determining the rate over two cardiac cycles (Fig. 9).

Fetal Dating

Accurate assessment of fetal age may impact triage and treatment decisions within the ED setting. In early pregnancy, age may be estimated by measuring the gestational sac or crown-rump–length. As pregnancy progresses, these methods become less accurate. In later pregnancy, biparietal diameter (BPD), abdominal circumference, or femur length may provide for assessment of fetal age.

Biparietal diameter is probably the most accurate single measurement (Fig. 12), and most US machines have calculation packages for determining fetal age based on these measurements.

Uterine Incarceration

As the uterus enlarges during pregnancy, it typically moves from the pelvic cavity into the abdominal cavity at 12 to 16 weeks of gestational age. However, in women with a retroverted uterus, the uterus

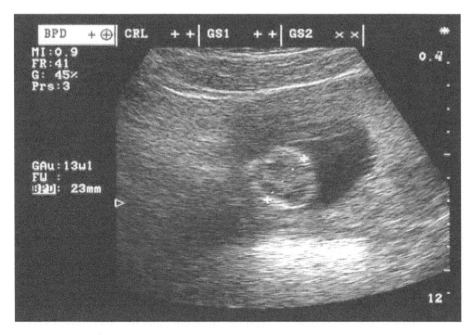

Figure 12
Fetal dating using biparietal diameter.

may fail to appropriately migrate. As the uterus enlarges, it may press on the urethra, preventing bladder emptying, which further obstructs the uterus from leaving the pelvis. Failure to recognize this condition may result in significant morbidity and mortality for both the mother and the fetus (52,53).

Sonographically, uterine incarceration appears as an enlarged bladder with a retroverted uterus inferior to the bladder, although diagnosis may be difficult and occasionally requires magnetic resonance imaging (54,55). Often, the simple placement of a foley catheter will empty the bladder and allow the uterus to rise out of the pelvis, though occasionally manipulation under anesthesia is required to reduce the uterus.

Placental Abruption

Placental abruption occurs in less than 1% of pregnancies but carries a high risk of preterm labor and fetal demise. Typically, this presents with significant pain and vaginal bleeding, and there is often a history of trauma. While US is the diagnostic test of choice and is fairly specific (approximately 93%), sensitivity remains poor (approximately 28%), and classic cases should proceed with management without US (56,57). When visualized, abruption appears as a hypoechoic hematoma posterior to the homogenous placenta.

Placenta Previa

Classically presenting with "painless vaginal bleeding," placenta previa is the leading cause of third trimester bleeding and occurs in 1 in 200 pregnancies. Prior cesarean section is the principal risk factor. While the placenta may cover the cervical os in early pregnancy, it typically moves away from this as the uterus enlarges. However, bleeding beyond the 24th week of gestation should prompt a US, which is reported to be 93% accurate for placenta previa (58,59). Patients with suspected previa should avoid manipulation of the cervix, including TVUS. Cesarean section is indicated if bleeding is severe or if the pregnancy is near-term.

PELVIC ULTRASOUND IN THE NONPREGNANT PATIENT

The nonpregnant female who presents to the ED with significant pelvic pain may be diagnostically difficult. The differential diagnosis ranges from benign causes such as menstrual cramps and ovarian cysts to more serious problems such as ovarian torsion and tubo-ovarian abscess. Bowel pathology, including appendicitis, may also present with pelvic pain.

Ovarian Cyst

The typical premenopausal ovary contains numerous follicular cysts of varying sizes (Fig. 13). Cysts over 2.5 cm are considered abnormal, although they are typically benign. A simple follicular cyst is round, anechoic, and thin-walled. During pregnancy, a corpus luteum cyst is often identified. These tend to have a slightly thicker but homogenous wall, and may reach sizes of up to 11 cm.

Hemorrhage may complicate both simple and corpus luteum cysts. Hemorrhagic cysts demonstrate internal debris that may progress to form septae over time (Fig. 14).

While most cysts are benign, large and complex cysts should be followed for resolution over time with serial US examinations.

Ovarian Torsion

Ovarian torsion is an uncommon but emergent cause of pelvic pain. Pain in torsion is typically severe, of sudden onset, and often involves vomiting, although presentations are nonspecific. Enlargement of the ovary due to cysts, induction of ovulation, or pregnancy are risk factors for torsion, which occurs more frequently on the right side. Approximately 25% of torsions occur during pregnancy, involving approximately 1 in 1800 pregnancies, typically between the 6th and 14th week of gestation (60).

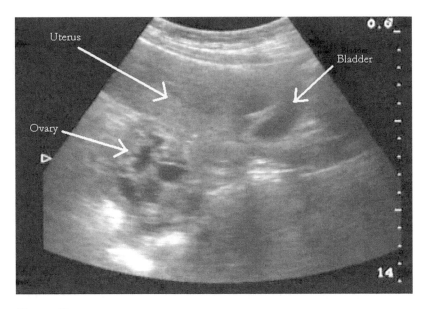

Figure 13
Ovary with follicles seen on transabdominal image.

    While variable in appearance, the torsed ovary is typically enlarged, with areas of hypoechogenicity (edema) as well as hyperechogenicity (hemorrhage). Classically, there are numerous peripheral follicles. Some

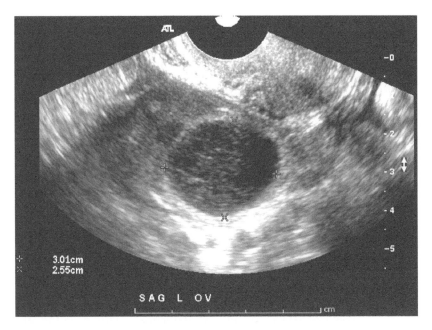

Figure 14
Hemorrhagic ovarian cyst. Note the debris seen inside of the cyst.

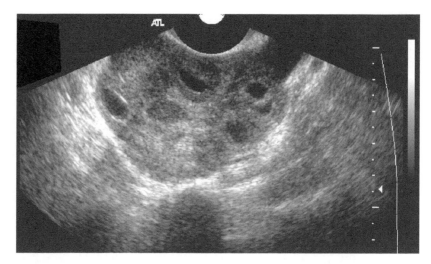

Figure 15
Enlarged ovary with peripheral follicles. This ovary was torsed, as definitively
demonstrated by the lack of flow in Figure 16.

degree of free fluid is typically seen in the pelvis (Fig. 15). The absence of
arterial flow on spectral Doppler is specific for torsion (Figs. 16 and 17),
although the overall sensitivity of US for torsion has been reported to be
as low as 40% (61).

Tubo-Ovarian Abscess

Approximately 5% of patients with pelvic inflammatory disease (PID)
progress to abscess formation; however, identification of abscess in
PID is important, because it may guide the clinician toward inpatient
treatment and surgical intervention. Classically the patient presents with
pelvic pain, vaginal discharge, and fever. While pregnancy is protective
for sexually transmitted disease, both PID and abscess may still occur
in these patients.

Sonographic findings of tubo-ovarian abscess include an irregular
matted appearance of the adnexae around the ovary, and may demonstrate hydrosalpinx or pyosalpinx.

FLUID IN THE PELVIS

Small amounts of fluid in the female pelvis are nonspecific and may be
normal. However, larger amounts of fluid may represent significant
hemorrhage from trauma, EUG, or ruptured ovarian cyst. Fluid may
spill from the pelvis into the abdominal cavity, or in the other direction.
When fluid is identified in the pelvis, a view of the abdomen for free fluid
should be included in the US examination.

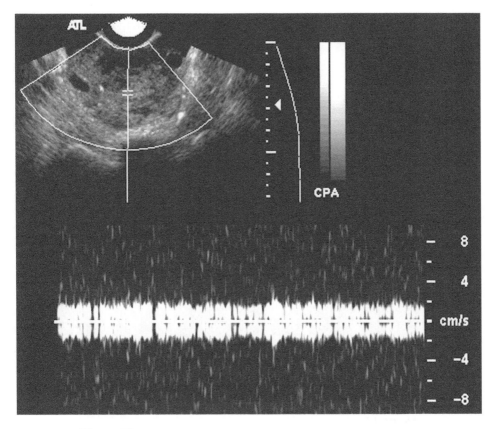

Figure 16
Spectral Doppler of a torsed ovary. The flow is monophasic, as contrasted to normal arterial flow in Figure 17.

Fluid in the Cul-de-sac

Also known as the "Pouch of Douglas," the rectouterine pouch or culde-sac is the most dependent portion of the female pelvis, and when free fluid is present in the pelvis it tends to collect here. Performance of a culdocentesis, a procedure rendered nearly obsolete by the proliferation of US (62–64), is intended to withdraw fluid from this area. On US, fluid in the cul-de-sac appears as an anechoic area posterior to the cervix with or without the presence of echogenic material (Figs. 5 and 18). Generally, it is subjectively rated as small, moderate, or large. Presence of a moderate anechoic fluid collection in the absence of IUP in symptomatic patients presents a relative risk for EUG of 5.2, while echogenic or large volume fluid presents a relative risk of 9.1 (65).

Anterior Uterovesicular Space

The space anterior to the uterus and between the uterus and bladder represents another potential space for fluid. This space typically only

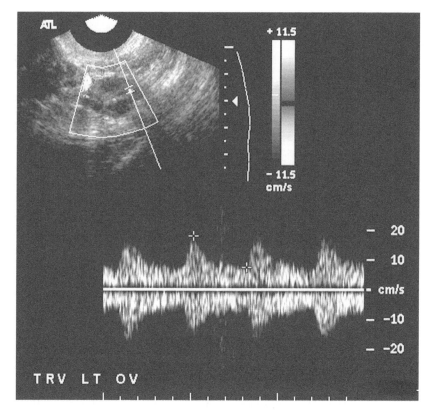

Figure 17
Normal spectral Doppler of the ovarian artery.

has fluid when there is a large amount of fluid in the pelvis. Fluid in this space is almost always abnormal.

Morrison's Pouch

The hepatorenal space, also known as a "Morrison's pouch," is the most sensitive sonographic area in the abdomen for detection of hemoperitoneum. Because rupture of EUG with significant bleeding will frequently cause fluid to collect in the peritoneal as well as pelvic spaces (66), it is recommended that the imaging of Morrison's pouch be incorporated as a routine part of the ultrasonographic examination for EUG.

The presence of fluid in the peritoneal space, positive β-hCG, and no IUP can be used as strong indirect evidence for an EUG (63). In a retrospective study of 37 ED patients who received operative intervention for ruptured EUG, the presence of a positive Morrison's pouch by EP-performed US was associated with a reduction in time to operative intervention of over three hours (from 322 minutes to 111 minutes) (4).

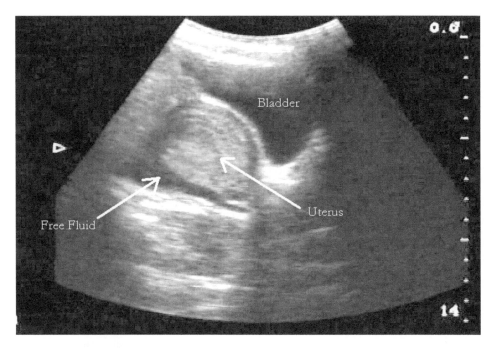

Figure 18
Transabdominal sagittal image, moderate-to-large amount of free fluid posterior to the uterus.

This view is typically obtained in a coronal plane at the right flank with a 2.5 to 5 MHz curvilinear transducer. Presence of an anechoic area between the liver and kidney on this view is indicative of at least 250 to 500 cc of fluid, usually indicating significant blood in the peritoneal space (Chapter 6).

REFERENCES

1. American College of Emergency Physicians. Clinical policy for the initial approach to patients presenting with a chief complaint of vaginal bleeding. Ann Emerg Med 1997; 29:435–458.
2. Durham B. Emergency medicine physicians saving time with ultrasound. Am J Emerg Med 1996; 14:309–313.
3. Shih CH. Effect of emergency physician-performed pelvic sonography on length of stay in the emergency department. Ann Emerg Med 1997; 29:348–351 [discussion 352].
4. Rodgerson JD, Heegaard WG, Plummer D, Hicks J, Clinton J, Sterner S. Emergency department right upper quadrant ultrasound is associated with a reduced time to diagnosis and treatment of ruptured ectopic pregnancies. Acad Emerg Med 2001; 8:331–336.
5. Filly RA. Ectopic pregnancy: the role of sonography. Radiology 1987; 162:661–668.
6. Pisarska MD, Carson SA, Buster JE. Ectopic pregnancy. Lancet 1998; 351:1115–1120.
7. Committee ACP, Clinical Policies Subcommittee on Early Pregnancy. American College of Emergency Physicians. Clinical policy: critical issues in the initial evaluation and management of patients presenting to the emergency department in early pregnancy. Ann Emerg Med 2003; 41:123–133.
8. Stovall TG, Kellerman AL, Ling FW, Buster JE. Emergency department diagnosis of ectopic pregnancy. Ann Emerg Med 1990; 19:1098–1103.
9. Barnhart K, Mennuti MT, Benjamin I, Jacobson S, Goodman D, Coutifaris C. Prompt diagnosis of ectopic pregnancy in an emergency department setting. Obstet Gynecol 1994; 84:1010–1015.
10. Abbott J, Emmans LS, Lowenstein SR. Ectopic pregnancy: ten common pitfalls in diagnosis. Am J Emerg Med 1990; 8:515–522.
11. Durston WE, Carl ML, Guerra W, Eaton A, Ackerson LM. Ultrasound availability in the evaluation of ectopic pregnancy in the ED: comparison of quality and cost-effectiveness with different approaches. Am J Emerg Med 2000; 18:408–417.
12. Robert W, DeVoe JHP. Simultaneous intrauterine and extrauterine pregnancy. Am J Obstet Gynecol 1948; 56:1119–1125.
13. Stephen R, Richards LES, Betsy D, Carlton. Heterotopic pregnancy: reappraisal of incidence. Am J Obstet Gynecol 1982; 142:928–930.
14. Thomsen T, Brown DF, Nadel ES. Abdominal pain in first trimester pregnancy. J Emerg Med 2003; 24:55–58.
15. O'Brien MC, Rutherford T. Misdiagnosis of bilateral ectopic pregnancies: a caveat about operator expertise in the use of transvaginal ultrasound. J Emerg Med 1993; 11:275–278.
16. Lipscomb GH, McCord ML, Stovall TG, Huff G, Portera SG, Ling FW. Predictors of success of methotrexate treatment in women with tubal ectopic pregnancies.[comment]. N Engl J Med Overseas Ed 1999; 341:1974–1978.
17. Alfthan H, Bjorses UM, Tiitinen A, Stenman UH. Specificity and detection limit of ten pregnancy tests. Scand J Clin Lab Invest Suppl 1993; 216:105–113.
18. Asch RH, Asch B, Asch G, Asch M, Bray R, Rojas FJ. Performance and sensitivity of modern home pregnancy tests. Int J Fertil 1988; 33:154, 157–158, 161.
19. Barnhart KT, Katz I, Hummel A, Gracia CR. Presumed diagnosis of ectopic pregnancy.[comment]. Obstet Gynecol 2002; 100:505–510.
20. Ankum WM, Van der Veen F, Hamerlynck JV, Lammes FB. Suspected ectopic pregnancy. What to do when human chorionic gonadotropin levels are below the discriminatory zone. J Reprod Med 1995; 40:525–528.
21. Mol BW, Hajenius PJ, Engelsbel S, Ankum WM, Van der Veen F, Hemrika DJ, Bossuyt PM. Serum human chorionic gonadotropin measurement in the diagnosis of ectopic pregnancy when transvaginal sonography is inconclusive. Fertil Steril 1998; 70:972–981.

22. Kadar N, DeVore G, Romero R. Discriminatory hCG zone: its use in the sonographic evaluation for ectopic pregnancy. Obstet Gynecol 1981; 58:156–161.
23. Chambers SE, Muir BB, Haddad NG. Ultrasound evaluation of ectopic pregnancy including correlation with human chorionic gonadotrophin levels. Br J Radiol 1990; 63:246–250.
24. Dart RG, Kaplan B, Cox C. Transvaginal ultrasound in patients with low beta-human chorionic gonadotropin values: how often is the study diagnostic? [comment]. Ann Emerg Med 1997; 30:135–140.
25. DiMarchi JM, Kosasa TS, Hale RW. What is the significance of the human chorionic gonadotropin value in ectopic pregnancy? Obstet Gynecol 1989; 74:851–855.
26. Kalinski MA, Guss DA. Hemorrhagic shock from a ruptured ectopic pregnancy in a patient with a negative urine pregnancy test result. Ann Emerg Med 2002; 40:102–105.
27. Kaplan BC, Dart RG, Moskos M, Kuligowska E, Chun B, Adel Hamid M, Northern K, Schmidt J, Kharwadkar A. Ectopic pregnancy: prospective study with improved diagnostic accuracy [comment]. Ann Emerg Med 1996; 28:10–17.
28. Barnhart KT, Simhan H, Kamelle SA. Diagnostic accuracy of ultrasound above and below the beta-hCG discriminatory zone.[comment]. Obstet Gynecol 1999; 94:583–587.
29. Barnhart K, Coutifaris C. Diagnosis of ectopic pregnancy.[comment]. Ann Emerg Med 1997; 29:295–296.
30. Dart RG, Mitterando J, Dart LM. Rate of change of serial beta-human chorionic gonadotropin values as a predictor of ectopic pregnancy in patients with indeterminate transvaginal ultrasound findings. Ann Emerg Med 1999; 34:703–710.
31. Barnhart KT, Katz I, Hummel A, Gracia CR. Presumed diagnosis of ectopic pregnancy. Obstet Gynecol 2002; 100:505–510.
32. Benacerraf B, Parker-Jones K, Schiff I. Decidual cast mimicking an intrauterine gestational sac and fetal pole in a patient with ectopic pregnancy. A case report. J Reprod Med 1984; 29:498–500.
33. Nyberg DA, Mack LA, Harvey D, Wang K. Value of the yolk sac in evaluating early pregnancies. J Ultrasound Med 1988; 7:129–135.
34. Bradley WG, Fiske CE, Filly RA. The double sac sign of early intrauterine pregnancy: use in exclusion of ectopic pregnancy. Radiology 1982; 143:223–226.
35. Nyberg DA, Laing FC, Filly RA, Uri-Simmons M, Jeffrey RB Jr. Ultrasonographic differentiation of the gestational sac of early intrauterine pregnancy from the pseudo-gestational sac of ectopic pregnancy. Radiology 1983; 146:755–759.
36. Lyons EAL, Clifford S, Dashefsky SM. The first trimester. Rumack CM, ed. Diagnostic Ultrasound. Vol. 2. St. Louis: Mosby, 1998:975–1011.
37. Albayram F, Hamper UM. First-trimester obstetric emergencies: spectrum of sonographic findings. J Clin Ultrasound 2002; 30:161–177.
38. Bennett GL, Bromley B, Lieberman E, Benacerraf BR. Subchorionic hemorrhage in first-trimester pregnancies: prediction of pregnancy outcome with sonography. Radiology 1996; 200:803–806.
39. Ball RH, Ade CM, Schoenborn JA, Crane JP. The clinical significance of ultransonographically detected subchorionic hemorrhages. Am J Obstet Gynecol 1002; 174:996–1002.
40. Fleischer AC, Pennell RG, McKee MS, Worrell JA, Keefe B, Herbert CM, Hill GA, Cartwright PS, Kepple DM. Ectopic pregnancy: features at transvaginal sonography. Radiology 1990; 174:375–378.
41. DeWitt C, Abbott J. Interstitial pregnancy: a potential for misdiagnosis of ectopic pregnancy with emergency department ultrasonography. Ann Emerg Med 2002; 40:106–109.
42. Binder DS. Use of ultrasonography in the emergency department: time for a reappraisal. [comment]. Ann Emerg Med 2003; 41:755–756.

43. Tarim E, Ulusan S, Kilicdag E, Yildirim T, Bagis T, Kuscu E. Angular pregnancy. J Obstet Gynaecol Res 2004; 30:377–379.
44. Maliha WE, Gonella P, Degnan EJ. Ruptured interstitial pregnancy presenting as an intrauterine pregnancy by ultrasound.[comment]. Ann Emerg Med 1991; 20:910–912.
45. Zorko MF. Rupture of cornual ectopic pregnancy after dilatation and curretage. Ann Emerg Med 1987; 16:808–810.
46. Chen GD, Lin MT, Lee MS. Diagnosis of interstitial pregnancy with sonography. J Clin Ultrasound 1994; 22:439–442.
47. de Boer CN, van Dongen PW, Willemsen WN, Klapwijk CW. Ultrasound diagnosis of interstitial pregnancy. Eur J Obstet Gynecol Reprod Biol 1992; 47:164–166.
48. Jauniaux E. Ultrasound diagnosis and follow-up of gestational trophoblastic disease. Ultrasound Obstet Gynecol 1998; 11:367–377.
49. Sairam S, Khare M, Michailidis G, Thilaganathan B. The role of ultrasound in the expectant management of early pregnancy loss. Ultrasound Obstet Gynecol 2001; 17:506–509.
50. Luise C, Jermy K, Collons WP, Bourne TH. Expectant management of incomplete, spontaneous first-trimester miscarriage: outcome according to initial ultrasound criteria and value of follow-up visits. Ultrasound Obstet Gynecol 2002; 19:580–582.
51. Sadan O, Golan A, Girtler O, Lurie S, Debby A, Sagiv R, Evron S, Glezerman M. Role of sonography in the diagnosis of retained products of conception. J Ultrasound Med 2004; 23:371–374.
52. Patterson E, Herd AM. Incarceration of the uterus in pregnancy. Am J Emerg Med 1997; 15:49–51.
53. Matsushita H, Kurabayashi T, Higashino M, Kojima Y, Takakuwa K, Tanaka K. Incarceration of the retroverted uterus at term gestation. Am J Perinatol 2004; 21:387–389.
54. van Beekhuizen HJ, Bodewes HW, Tepe EM, Oosterbaan HP, Kruitwagen R, Nijland R. Role of magnetic resonance imaging in the diagnosis of incarceration of the gravid uterus. Obstet Gynecol 1134; 102:1134–1137.
55. Chen LL, Goldstein RB. Case 9. Incarcerated uterus. J Ultrasound Med 2002; 21:613–614.
56. Moore C, Promes SB. Ultrasound in pregnancy. Emerg Med Clin North Am 2004; 22:697–722.
57. Glantz C, Purnell L. Clinical utility of sonography in the diagnosis and treatment of placental abruption. J Ultrasound Med 2002; 21:837–840.
58. Baron F, Hill WC. Placenta previa, placenta abruptio. Clin Obstet Gynecol 1998; 41:527–532.
59. Hudon L, Belfort MA, Broome DR. Diagnosis and management of placenta percreta: a review. Obstet Gynecol Surv 1998; 53:509–517.
60. Webb EM, Green GE, Scoutt LM. Adnexal mass with pelvic pain. Radiol Clin North Am 2004; 42:329–348.
61. Pena JE, Ufberg D, Cooney N, Denis AL. Usefulness of Doppler sonography in the diagnosis of ovarian torsion.[see comment]. Fertil Steril 2000; 73(5):1047–1050.
62. Stovall TG, Ling FW. Ectopic pregnancy. Diagnostic and therapeutic algorithms minimizing surgical intervention. J Reprod Med 1993; 38:807–812.
63. Atri M, Valenti DA, Bret PM, Gillett P. Effect of transvaginal sonography on the use of invasive procedures for evaluating patients with a clinical diagnosis of ectopic pregnancy. J Clin Ultrasound 2003; 31:1–8.
64. Kim DS, Chung SR, Park MI, Kim YP. Comparative review of diagnostic accuracy in tubal pregnancy: a 14-year survey of 1040 cases. Obstet Gynecol 1987; 70:547–554.
65. Dart R, McLean SA, Dart L. Isolated fluid in the cul-de-sac: how well does it predict ectopic pregnancy? Am J Emerg Med 2002; 20:1–4.
66. Popat RU, Adams CP. Diagnosis of ruptured ectopic pregnancy by bedside ultrasonography. J Emerg Med 2002; 22:409–410.

8
Basic Cardiac Echo

Paul Mayo
Pulmonary and Critical Care Medicine, Beth Israel Medical Center, New York, New York, U.S.A.

INTRODUCTION

This chapter will provide an overview of echocardiography for the noncardiologist, beginning with a review of some technical issues related to the physics of echocardiography followed by a summary of the constituent parts of the echocardiographic examination. Following will be a discussion of challenges related to achieving competence in the field as a noncardiologist and, finally, some clinical applications of echocardiography that are of relevance to the noncardiologist.

TECHNICAL ISSUES

Echocardiography utilizes ultrasound (US) waves in identical fashion to diagnostic sonography elsewhere in the body. In fact, an echocardiography machine can be used effectively for abdominal and general thoracic sonography, as the physical principles of echocardiography are similar to general sonography. A detailed discussion of the physics of diagnostic ultrasonography may be found elsewhere in this text.

Echocardiography has technical problems that relate to the position of the heart within the thorax. Ribs block transmission of US waves. For this reason, echocardiographic transducers are small-size sector type to permit imaging through intercostal spaces. If possible, the patient should be imaged with the left arm abducted, in order to increase left intercostal space size. Air-filled lung also blocks transmission of US. Positioning the patient properly is important in obtaining good image quality. The left lateral decubitus position brings the heart against the chest wall without intervening lung and is a favored position when examining the heart from the apex. Patients on ventilatory support, particularly if on positive end expiratory pressure (PEEP) or with emphysema, are difficult to study as an air-filled lung may block image acquisition during ventilator cycling. Image quality may be poor on patients who are very muscular or obese;

and extensive chest wounds, dressings, and difficulty in positioning the patient who is critically ill may make trans-thoracic echocardiography (TTE) difficult. The subcostal window may be useful, but trans-esophageal echocardiography (TEE) remains an alternative in the difficult-to-image patient. The presence of a large pleural effusion or densely consolidated lung should be seen as an opportunity to perform TTE from points on the thorax ordinarily blocked by aerated lung, as US transmission may be quite adequate in this circumstance.

The best resolution of a sonographic interface occurs if the sonogram beam is perpendicular to the interface of interest. The opposite applies for Doppler measurement, where the Doppler interrogation is best accomplished with the sonogram beam oriented parallel to blood flow. Echocardiographic technique must take these issues into consideration. Another issue is that structures that are far away from the transducer require a lower frequency transducer; this reduces resolution and frame rate. The echocardiographer must become proficient in optimizing machine settings and transducer position to obtain adequate image quality and Doppler signal.

There are many different types of two-dimensional (2D) image and Doppler artifacts that are characteristic of diagnostic ultrasonography, but not peculiar to echocardiography. The echocardiographer must be thoroughly familiar with these many artifacts. An artifact that is peculiar to 2D echocardiography relates to the fact that the heart is a highly mobile organ. As it contracts, it can move very vigorously in the chest. Translational, rotational, and torsional movement of the heart may be misinterpreted as reflecting contractile function or vice versa. Distinguishing between a movement artifact of this type and actual cardiac contraction is a challenge that can only be surmounted with experience.

THE COMPLETE ECHOCARDIOGRAM

A complete TTE will generally include specific 2D anatomic views and a comprehensive Doppler examination. Equivalent anatomic views and Doppler measurements are sought when performing TEE. These standard anatomic views are well summarized in position statements by the American Society of Echocardiography (ASE) (1–3). They should be completely familiar to the echocardiographer. Every complete echocardiogram should include an attempt at these well-defined anatomic views. They typically include the parasternal long axis, the right ventricular inflow, the right ventricular outflow, the parasternal short axis aortic valve level, the parasternal short axis mid-left ventricular level, the apical four chamber, the apical two chamber, the apical three chamber, and the subcostal view. Specialized views may be added to the standard 2D examination as needed such as suprasternal for TTE and the pulmonary venous inflow and deep gastric views for the TEE. The TEE is especially useful for imaging the aorta and the posterior cardiac structures. The

TEE transducer is of higher frequency than that used for TTE. This permits excellent resolution of posterior cardiac anatomy but sacrifices penetration. Anterior cardiac structures are better imaged with TTE, as there is better penetration with a lower frequency transducer than with the TEE probe.

Each of the standard views permits optimal visualization of various parts of the heart, their sum permitting the examiner to achieve a complete assessment of anatomy and function. The 2D study attempts to assess overall left and right ventricular function, segmental wall function, chamber size, wall thickness, valvular anatomy and function, the pericardium, and the presence or absence of other disease processes such as vegetation, thrombus, cardiac masses, or congenital heart disease. The 2D examination also permits quantitative measurement of ejection fraction and stroke volume.

A comprehensive TTE and TEE includes a full Doppler study. Doppler echocardiography allows measurement of blood velocity as it flows through the heart and adjacent blood vessels. Through application of the simplified Bernoulli equation, blood flow velocity through cardiac chambers and across valves can be converted to a pressure gradient. In addition, measurement of stroke volume is straightforward with Doppler ultrasonography. This permits a wide variety of both qualitative and quantitative hemodynamic measurements to be made both with TTE and TEE. The list of possible measurements that can be made is extensive and depends on the clinical needs of the study, the ingenuity of the examiner, and the time available for study.

Examples of Doppler measurements easily obtained both by TTE or TEE include the following:

1. *Measurement of diastolic dysfunction*: For the left ventricle, this is achieved by analysis of mitral valve inflow pattern and pulmonary venous inflow (4). Right-sided diastolic function is assessed by Doppler measurement of tricuspid inflow and hepatic venous flow pattern. Tissue Doppler imaging and left ventricular color M-mode flow velocity propagation are also useful (5).

2. *Measurement of intracardiac pressures*: The presence of valvular regurgitation allows measurement of the velocity and therefore the pressure gradient existing across the affected valve, using the modified Bernoulli equation. If the chamber pressure on one side of the valve is known, the measured pressure gradient across the valve allows calculation of the pressure in the adjacent chamber. For example, if right atrial pressure is known and the velocity of a tricuspid regurgitation jet is measured by Doppler; the transvalvular pressure gradient so derived is added to the right atrial pressure to give a right ventricular systolic pressure. Right ventricular systolic pressure is equal to the pulmonary artery systolic pressure, in the absence of pulmonic valve stenosis. This general principle can be used for accurate measurement of many

intracardiac pressures. The Doppler examiner always hopes for significant valvular regurgitation, as this permits assessment of intracardiac pressures.

3. *Quantitative measurement of stroke volume*: This is usually performed at the left ventricular outflow tract, though Doppler-derived stroke volume can be measured at several different points in the heart. Knowledge of stroke volume then allows calculation of values for indexed stroke volume, cardiac output, and vascular resistance measurements. Assessment of ventricular function can also be made by measurement of dP/dt of both ventricles (6,7) provided the mitral or tricuspid regurgitation is present.

4. *Qualitative estimate of pulmonary artery occlusion pressure*: This is achieved by analysis of pulmonary venous and mitral valve inflow Doppler waveforms (8). Color M-mode flow velocity propagation of left ventricular inflow (9) may be used to supplement these measurements, as well as tissue Doppler of the mitral annulus when combined with standard mitral inflow measurement (10).

5. *Quantitative analysis of valvular stenosis and regurgitation*: By measurement of stroke volume and application of the continuity equation, cross-sectional valve area, regurgitant fraction, regurgitant volume, and effective regurgitant orifice measurements can be made in order to quantitate valvular dysfunction. Proximal isovelocity surface area method is an alternative method.

6. *Identification of left ventricular systolic outflow obstruction*: Left ventricular systolic outflow obstruction is often first suspected by findings on two-dimensional echocardiography. Doppler examination permits confirmation of this important entity.

7. *Qualitative assessment of blood flow by color flow imaging*: Color flow imaging allows qualitative analysis of valvular regurgitation, as well as a variety of abnormal blood flow velocity patterns associated with cardiac pathology. The entry-level echocardiographer may find it especially attractive due to its intuitively obvious image pattern. Its strength is in its ease of use, while its weakness lies in its qualitative nature and subjective interpretation. The reader is reminded that color flow Doppler does not actually reflect blood flow but the velocity of blood flow; the images should not be interpreted as equivalent to angiographic images.

8. *Diagnosis of pericardial tamponade and constriction*: Analysis of mitral valve, pulmonary venous, tricuspid valve, and hepatic venous flow patterns permit diagnosis of this pathophysiology.

The above list of Doppler measurements is by no means complete. I include the list to emphasize to the entry-level practitioner the importance of Doppler study in echocardiography. Doppler and 2D echocardiography should be viewed as complementary. It is straightforward in its mastery and should be an integral part of every comprehensive TTE and TEE.

M-mode echocardiography is of historic interest, but it may not be necessary as part of a standard examination with a modern machine. Its main utility relates to its very high sampling rate (1600 Hz is typical), which permits resolution of very rapidly moving cardiac structures. The reader is recommended to it as an optional field of study. Knowledge of M-mode will certainly improve the reader's understanding of 2D images.

Should every echocardiogram include all the standard 2D views, a comprehensive Doppler study, and even M-mode measurements? Many examinations are performed by highly trained sonography technicians and reviewed later in a reading room by the interpreting cardiologist who often will never see the patient and who has minimal knowledge of the actual clinical situation. This favors an approach requiring a comprehensive examination in all cases. Reimbursement issues are also a consideration that drives the concept that all examinations must be of a comprehensive nature. An alternative approach is to perform limited studies that are directed by the clinical situation at hand. This might apply in the case of a patient who has had an initial comprehensive exam, but whose clinical course is rapidly changing. Repeated re-examination in order to guide therapy in the critically ill will often be of a directed but limited type. The clinician who is in charge of the patient would be the appropriate echocardiographer in this situation, rather than a technician and clinically uninvolved offline reader. However, the clinician who uses echocardiography in this fashion must clearly be knowledgeable concerning the comprehensive echocardiogram. This leads the discussion to the complex issues of how to obtain training and achieve competence in echocardiography as a noncardiologist.

TRAINING, COMPETENCE, AND CERTIFICATION ISSUES

In the United States, echocardiography is considered an integral part of the subspecialty of cardiology. Historically, cardiologists from its inception developed the field. Training in echocardiography is a required part of cardiology fellowship training. In both academic- and community-based practice, it is uncommon to find any but cardiologists who perform echocardiography. The situation is analogous to that in sonography, which is very much dominated by the specialty of radiology. Powerful forces combine to perpetuate the dominance of echocardiography by cardiologists. These include issues related to simple tradition, lack of access to training for noncardiologists, powerful economic prerogatives, and political control issues. An exception to this dominance is in the field of intraoperative TEE, where cardiac anesthesiologists have established a niche for themselves that includes a formal certification process under the aegis of the ASE (11).

The situation is different elsewhere in the world. In Europe and Asia, both general sonography and echocardiography are considered the province of any clinician who is interested in the field. In Germany and Japan, for example, training in sonography and echocardiography is often part of general internal medicine residency training and is incorporated as needed into subspecialty training as well. In France, intensivists are often highly trained echocardiographers as reflected in their impressive research in this area. Our colleagues abroad have a more inclusive approach and regard sonography and echocardiography as being for the benefit of patient care rather than as the exclusive domain of any particular specialty. The reality is that echocardiography is a field that can be mastered by any interested clinician irrespective of specialty, provided the individual is able to make the commitment to learning the skill.

In 2003, the American College of Cardiology (ACC), the American Heart Association (AHA), and the American College of Physicians-American Society of Internal Medicine published the ACC/AHA Clinical Competence Statement on Echocardiography (The Statement) (12). The report was developed in collaboration with other relevant organizations including the ASE. The Statement is the definitive opinion on the subject, and the reader may use it as a road map to follow in developing competence in the field. I will review some important parts of The Statement and encourage the reader to read it in detail.

The Statement posits that there are several definable aspects to being a skilled echocardiographer. These include basic knowledge, cognitive requirements, training requirements, proof of competence, and maintenance of competence.

The Statement summarizes the factual knowledge required to become a skilled echocardiographer as follows:

1. *Basic knowledge of ultrasound physics*: This knowledge is readily available in standard texts on echocardiography.
2. *Technical aspects of the examination*: The Statement emphasizes that the echocardiographers must have the personal capacity to perform all aspects of the examination themselves. It is unacceptable to rely on a technician for this purpose. This requires complete mastery of the controls of the machine as well as a high-level of skill in transducer manipulation. The latter is an underappreciated part of training. From the point of view of the noncardiologist, the need to be highly competent in all aspects of image and Doppler acquisition cannot be overemphasized. This is especially true in the intensive care unit, as the physician will perform the actual examination without technician support and make clinical decisions based on the results.
3. *Anatomy and physiology*: The Statement emphasizes that the trainee must have a strong working knowledge of cardiac anatomy and physiology in order to apply echocardiographic results to the clinical context. This is one area where cardiologists have a distinct advantage, as their training background

and everyday clinical activity results in a high-level of familiarity with these subjects. The noncardiologist will need to study the subject intensively.

4. *Recognition of simple and complex pathology*: This aspect of training requires the careful interpretation of numerous studies under the supervision of a skilled echocardiographer-teacher.

In addition to the basic knowledge required for echocardiography, The Statement lists the cognitive skills required for competence in TTE and TEE, as well as other more specialized aspects of the field. The Statement then moves to an issue of particular interest to the noncardiologist—training requirements for the performance and interpretation of both TTE and TEE. These are summarized in Tables 1 and 2. The Statement defines three skill levels. The numerical requirements should be seen as minimum numbers, and performance and interpretation imply training in the basic knowledge and cognitive skills listed above. Training requirements are different from proof of competence. The Statement sets down guidelines for proof of competence. The Statement does not require a physician to be a subspecialist in cardiology in order to fulfill proof of competence. Any physician who can fulfill the training requirements of The Statement can prove competence in TTE and/or TEE. The clinician must have performed and interpreted the requisite number of studies under appropriate supervision, and then receive a letter or certificate from the training supervisor.

Table 1
Training Requirements for Performance and Interpretation of Adult Transthoracic Echocardiography

	Cumulative duration of training	Minimum total number of examinations performed	Minimum number of examinations interpreted
Level 1	3 months	75	150
Level 2	6 months	150 (75 additional)	300 (150 additional)
Level 3	12 months	300 (150 additional)	750 (450 additional)

Table 2
Training Requirements for Performance and Interpretation of TEE

Component	Objective	Approximate case load
General transthoracic echo, Level 2	Background knowledge and skills	300 interpreted 150 performed
Esophageal intubation	TBE probe introduction	25
TEE examinations	Skills in performance and interpretation	50

The noncardiologist faces the challenge of arranging this training and developing a close working relationship with a teaching echocardiographer who will generally be a level 3 echocardiographer.

There is a parallel track to prove competence in TTE and TEE. The Statement will also accept as proof of competence National Board of Echocardiography (NBE) certification. This alternate method is difficult for the noncardiologist to achieve. The NBE was founded in 1998 to establish criteria for special competence in Adult Echocardiography. Its requirements (13) include successful passing of a written board examination known as the ASCeXAM as well as fulfillment of training requirements established by the NBE. These requirements are very similar to those of The Statement although with certain provisos. The NBE has decided that past June 30, 2005, only cardiologists will be offered certification by the NBE. Before that time, NBE requirements for noncardiologists have been very restrictive, and so it has been difficult to achieve NBE certification in any case. Fortunately, The Statement presents an alternative policy that recognizes that noncardiologists may establish competence in the field without NBE certification. In doing so, it is stating the obvious; there is nothing intrinsic to echocardiography that requires full training in the subspecialty of cardiology.

The Statement includes discussion on the maintenance of competence for both TTE and TEE. In addition, it includes recommendations related to echocardiography using hand-carried ultrasound (HCU) devices. The Statement concludes that users of HCU devices should have, at the minimum, a level 1 training. The modern HCU device is low cost with excellent image quality and may be equipped with full Doppler capability. Image quality and Doppler measurement are now equivalent to the larger, standard sonographic machines (14). Their ease of use is seductive to the unsophisticated clinician, and the reader should heed the caution of The Statement: "HCU technology may yield ... incomplete, inadequate, or inaccurate information." The HCU should not be interpreted "as a license for untrained individuals to use poor imaging techniques that will result in inaccurate diagnosis" (12).

Another approach to training in echocardiography is for the clinician to focus training effort on the parts of the examination that have clinical relevance to their practice. The Statement implicitly rejects this option. For example, it suggests that users of the HCU be at least level 1. On the other hand, consensus statement by emergency medicine authorities defines less stringent training requirements (15). The ASE warns of the risks of inadequate training as follows: "However, even ... apparently straight forward conditions may be misdiagnosed or misinterpreted by persons who have insufficient training. Cardiac ultrasonography, even for 'quick look' or 'limited' examinations, requires substantial training to avoid diagnostic errors .... A disservice may result if those performing the definitive interpretation do not have appropriate skills and experience" (16). Several studies demonstrate that clinicians can become competent in specific parts of the TTE (17,18) and TEE examination (19) with minimal training. In ICU work, echocardiograhic examination may often be quite limited, and one could argue that an intensivist has no need to learn about obscure echocardiographic findings of congenital heart disease or nuanced Doppler measurements of valvular heart disease. Manasia et al. (54), have shown that intensivists can learn to perform a limited or "goal directed" TEE, and that this type of training has clinical utility in the management of the critically ill.

For those who seek advanced training in echocardiography, my own advice is that the noncardiologist would do well to follow The Statement closely. This will protect the patient, maintain the integrity of the clinician, and avoid issues of competence that may shadow the noncardiologist. Whether to achieve level 1 or level 2 training is a decision related to the needs of the trainee.

What specific steps should the noncardiologist take to obtain training? I have the following specific suggestions.

1. Many hours of serious study is required to acquire the knowledge base needed for TTE and TEE. Two excellent entry-level texts are standard in the field (20,21). I strongly recommend careful study of both, as they are complementary. In addition, purchase of a definitive reference text is important. The two classics in the field are very comprehensive but lack discussion of recent advances in the field (22,23). A more recent text by Otto (24) is now available. Programmatic problem-oriented texts are useful for Doppler training. A high quality anatomic heart model is very useful for training purposes (Denoyer-Geppert Chicago, Illinois, U.S.). To demonstrate definitive mastery of the knowledge base of the field, I would strongly advise the trainee who seeks advanced training to take the NBE sponsored board examination. The ASCeXAM (25) is conducted annually in June, and is a very challenging examination. Applications may be obtained from the ASE website (13). The pass rate for cardiologists is approximately 65% and 40% for noncardiologists. Though The Statement does not require it for proof of competence, the noncardiologist should consider taking it; as it offers objective proof of capability to those who might question otherwise. Interestingly, only a small proportion of cardiologists have taken the ASCeXAM.

2. To achieve a high level of skill with the transducer and machine setup, the trainee will need to personally perform a large number of examinations. Echocardiograhic technicians are highly skilled in all aspects of image acquisition and are an excellent learning resource. In addition, much can be learned from a skilled physician echocardiographer. Image acquisition requires constant practice, and this is best accomplished if the trainee has complete control of an echocardiography machine. The cost of a good quality sonogram machine with full Doppler capability is substantial. However, if the machine is multipurpose, the per-study cost is low. In a busy ICU, a sonogram machine that

is used for echocardiography, abdominal and pleural sonography, and vascular imaging may be used several thousand times per year. The main ongoing operating cost remains the renewal of a comprehensive warranty; the cost of machine operation is otherwise negligible and includes those of printer paper, sonographic gel, and long term data storage.

3. Image interpretation requires reviewing and interpreting a large number of studies under the direct supervision of a skilled teaching echocardiographer. This requires regular attendance in the echocardiogram reading room, as well as bedside teaching. This is not a skill amenable to self-teaching. All cardiology fellows are trained in this fashion, and the noncardiologist should seek no alternative. The main issue is one of cross specialty relations. Does the cardiologist have a problem with training a noncardiologist? This is an issue that can only be settled by the individuals involved. From a practical point of view, training is easily achieved during fellowship training. A typical pulmonary critical care fellowship will include many months of elective time. Goodwill being present, the interested trainee can simply arrange to enter the echocardiographic training sequence in parallel with cardiology fellows. Just as they are trained, so can a fellow from an outside service be trained with similar results. The principles of training for the noncardiologist who is already attending are the same. The challenge is to find a committed teacher as well as to find the time required to become skilled at image interpretation. Image interpretation requires a close teaching relationship as well reading a large number of examinations. As the trainee becomes more proficient at reading, other resources are available to improve image interpretation. The ACC and ASE have web sites that regularly feature challenging cases for interpretation. Most echocardiographic departments keep teaching files that can be reviewed as unknown cases by the trainee. Review courses and commercially available case collections are valuable learning tools as well. I would emphasize the absolute primacy of finding a good mentor, as well as the need to review a large number of varied examinations.

CLINICAL APPLICATIONS OF ECHOCARDIOGRAPHY BY THE NONCARDIOLOGIST

Why might a noncardiologist seek training in a field that is so completely identified with cardiology? I envision two groups of clinicians with this interest. Internists or family practice clinicians who practice in geographic areas where competent cardiologists cannot provide echocardiography services would have a natural interest in this field. This might occur in medically underserved areas. Competent cardiologists are widely dispersed in the United States, so this group of clinicians must be relatively small. They should seek level 2 training, as I would assume they would be interpreting echocardiograms as the definitive reader. In essence, this group would deliver the same service as a cardiologist who is skilled in the field. Another group of clinicians who would have interest in developing competence in diagnostic echocardiography are critical care specialists. The fulltime intensivist who is involved in actual hands-on management of the critically ill might be particularly interested in acquiring the skill.

Conceptually, echocardiography has obvious applications in ICU. Severe hemodynamic failure is a common presentation of critical illness, and echocardiography is an effective means to render diagnosis. Respiratory failure is another common presentation of critical illness. Cardiac dysfunction may be the cause of respiratory failure, and echocardiography permits prompt assessment of this important possibility. Frequently, several simultaneous pathophysiological pathways may be present, and echocardiography may help to distinguish their contribution. Anatomic and functional assessments are achieved readily with 2D study, while Doppler echocardiography allows detailed hemodynamic assessment. Beyond its utility in rapid diagnosis, echocardiography may be helpful in guiding the ongoing therapy of the critically ill.

The concept of echocardiography as a guide to ongoing therapy derives directly from its use by cardiac anesthesiologists. Standard practice in this field is to leave a TEE probe in place throughout an open-heart procedure. This allows real-time assessment of hemodynamics, contractile function, and volume status of the heart. TEE is ideally suited to this task, as the probe can be left in unobtrusively for several hours. TTE can only be performed intermittently, and is therefore best suited for initial diagnostic study and intermittent assessment for development of disease and response to therapy.

Many groups have reported on the utility and safety of TEE in the ICU (26–36). It appears to be well tolerated and to give clinically useful information. Of particular interest to the noncardiologist is the paper by Colreavy et al. (37,38), which describes the work of three intensivists who obtained advanced training in TEE. Benjamin et al. (19) also describe successful training of intensivists in limited TEE study with positive results. Echocardiography has some specific applications in the ICU that deserve specific mention. TEE is useful in the immediate diagnosis of central pulmonary embolism (39,40). Both TTE and TEE are useful in the assessment of right heart function in the critically ill (41,42). TTE is the best means of guiding pericardiocentesis (43). Both TTE and TEE permit qualitative assessment of left atrial pressures (44,45). TEE can assess volume status of the left ventricle and predict response to volume challenge in shock states (46–48). Respiratory pulse pressure variation can be detected by Doppler analysis (49,50). A strong argument can be made that the combination of echocardiography with respiratory pulse pressure variation has rendered the pulmonary artery catheter obsolete technology.

Both TTE and TEE have application in the ICU. As expected, several studies report that TEE may give information not obtainable with

TTE. However, TTE is often sufficient in the critically ill. Cook et al. (51) report patient characteristics that make TTE difficult to perform in the surgical ICU. These include PEEP above 15 cm H_2O, weight-gain > 10% of admission weight, and the presence of chest tubes. Most of the descriptive literature in echocardiography in the ICU reports on the use of TEE. In my experience, TTE often suffices. The choice of initial study must be determined by the clinical situation. Certain patients simply cannot be imaged with TTE. Chest wounds, surgical dressings, massive edema, or massive obesity are obvious indications that the critically ill patient is best imaged with TEE. Suspicion of aortic pathology, pulmonary embolism, or a postcardiotomy compressive localized pericardial effusion would dictate initial TEE. In general, medical ICU patients are good candidates for initial TTE. Surgical ICU patients, particularly postcardiac surgery cases, are often best imaged with TEE. For the intensivist entering the field, I would recommend developing proficiency in both TTE and TEE, as they are complementary modalities. For the medical intensivist, TTE training should have priority. From a practical standpoint, TEE probes are expensive, and have somewhat limited view of anterior cardiac structures. They also require special cleaning. Nonintubated patients who are critically ill with unstable respiratory status are not safe candidates for the sedation and airway complications that are intrinsic to TEE. The most appropriate candidate for TEE in the critically ill is the patient who has a technically inadequate TTE, who is intubated on a ventilator, and who has clear indication for the study. As the major risk of TEE is related to airway complication, once the patient is intubated and on a mechanical ventilator, the procedure is low risk. To facilitate introduction of the probe in patients who have an endotracheal tube in place, the TEE probe may be inserted under direct vision using a standard laryngoscopy blade. In selected patients, the probe may be left in place for a time in order to follow response and to guide acute resuscitation. Ideally, the reader will seek competence in both TTE and TEE, but will find that the former is very often quite adequate. It is often difficult to perform a sufficient number of TEEs for training purposes. I have found that a cooperative relationship with a competent cardiac anesthesiologist is a useful means of obtaining experience with TEE.

Who should receive an echocardiogram in the ICU? My approach is to perform a complete echocardiogram on all critically ill patients with significant hemodynamic failure and in those who have respiratory failure of ambiguous origin or where there is reasonable chance of coexisting heart disease. Unless there is indication for immediate TEE, TTE is the best initial approach. The test is safe, low cost, and uses equipment that has many other applications in the ICU. It can be tied into an approach that uses general screening ultrasonography in the critically ill (52). The main drawback that I encounter relates to the time required, particularly when using echocardiography for ongoing reassessment of the progression of disease and response to therapy. Vieillard-Baron et al. (53) use echocardiography as a primary diagnostic modality in the critically ill with hemodynamic instability. This group has fully integrated echocardiography into their ICU practice. Their sophisticated use of echocardiography is a paradigm for all intensivists to follow and should dispel any doubt as to the utility of echocardiography in the ICU. As echocardiography has such obvious application in the ICU, a strong argument can be made that training in the modality should be a routine part of critical care fellowship training.

CONCLUSION

In summary, echocardiography is a technique that provides important information regarding the anatomy and physiology of the heart. It is a skill that can be mastered by noncardiologists. There is a well-defined set of skills that are required to achieve competence in the field. Echocardiography has special application in the diagnosis and treatment of the critically ill, and intensivists may wish to consider introducing it into their clinical practice.

REFERENCES

1. Henry WL, DeMaria A, Gramiak R, King DL, Kisslo JA, Popp RL, Sahn DJ, Schiller NB, Tajik A, Teichholz LE, et al. Report of the American Society of Echocardiography Committee on the nomenclature and standards in two-dimensional echocardiography, 1980. http://asecho.org/Guidelines_Documents/body_guidelines_and_documents.php.
2. Schiller NB, Maurer G, Ritter SB, Armstrong WF, Crawford M, Spotnitz H, Cahalan M, Quinones M, Meltzer R, Feinstein S, et al. Transesophageal echocardiography. J Am Soc Echocardiogr 1989; 2:354–357.
3. Shanewise JS, Cheung AT, Aronson S, Stewart WJ, Weiss RL, Mark JB, Savage RM, Sears-Rogan P, Mathew JP, Quinones MA, et al. ASE/SCA guidelines for performing a comprehensive intraoperative multiplane transesophageal echocardiography examination: recommendations of the American Society of Echocardiography Council for intraoperative echocardiography and the Society of Cardiovascular Anesthesiologists task force for certification in perioperative transesophageal echocardiography. J Am Soc Echocardiogr 1999; 12:884–900.
4. Khouri SJ, Maly GT, Suh DD, Walsh TE. A practical approach to the echocardiographic evaluation of diastolic function. J Am Soc Echocardiogr 2004; 17:290–297.
5. Garcia MJ, Thomas JD, Klein AL. New Doppler echocardiographic applications for the study of diastolic function. J Am Coll Cardiol 1998; 32:865–875.
6. Imanishi T, Nakatani S, Yamada S, Nakanishi N, Beppu S, Nagata S, Miyatake K. Validation of continuous wave Doppler-determined right ventricular peak positive and negative dp/dt: effect of right atrial pressure on measurement. J Am Coll Cardiol 1994; 23:1638–1643.
7. Chung N, Nishimura RA, Holmes DR Jr, Tajik AJ. Measurement of left ventricular dp/dt by simultaneous Doppler echocardiography and cardiac catheterization. J Am Soc Echocardiogr 1992; 5:147–152.
8. Appleton CP, Galloway JM, Gonzalez MS, Gaballa M, Basnight MA. Estimation of left ventricular filling pressures using two-dimensional and Doppler echocardiography in adult patients with cardiac disease: additional value of analyzing left atrial size, left atrial ejection fraction and the difference in duration of pulmonary venous and mitral flow velocity at atrial contraction. J Am Coll Cardiol 1993; 22:1972–1982.
9. Garcia MJ, Ares MA, Asher C, Rodriguez L, Vandervoort P, Thomas JD. Color M-mode flow velocity propagation: an index of early left ventricular filling that combined with pulsed Doppler peak E velocity may predict capillary wedge pressure. J Am Coll Cardiol 1997; 29:448–454.
10. Ommen SR, Nishimura RA, Appleton CP, Miller FA, Oh JK, Redfield MM, Tajik AJ. Clinical utility of Doppler echocardiography and tissue Doppler imaging in the estimation of left ventricular filling pressures: a comparative simultaneous Doppler-catheterization study. Circulation 2000; 102:1788–1794.
11. Cahalan MK, Stewart W, Pearlman A, Goldman M, Sears-Rogan P, Abel M, Russell I, Shanewise J, Troianos C. American Society of Echocardiography and Society of Cardiovascular Anesthesiologists task force guidelines for training in perioperative echocardiography. J Amer Soc Echocardiogr 2002; 15:647–652.
12. Quinones MA, Douglas PS, Foster E, Gorcsan J III, Lewis JF, Pearlman AS, Rychik J, Salcedo EE, Seward JB, Stevenson JG, et al. ACC/AHA Clinical competence statement on echocardiography. J Am Coll Cardiol 2003; 41:687–708.
13. Application for 2004 Examination of Special Competence in Adult Echocardiography and Certification in Echocardiography. http://www.echoboards.org/pte/boardcertapp04.pdf.
14. Borges AC, Knebel F, Walde T, Sanad W, Baumann G. Diagnostic accuracy of new handheld echocardiography with Doppler and harmonic imaging properties. J Amer Soc Echocardiogr 2004; 17:234–238.

15. Heller MB, Mandavia D, Tayal VS, Cardenas EE, Lambert MJ, Mateer J, Melanson SW, Peimann NP, Plummer DW, Stahmer SA. Residency training in emergency ultrasound: fulfilling the mandate. Acad Emerg Med 2002; 9:835—839.
16. Stewart WJ, Douglas PS, Sagar K, Seward JB, Armstrong WF, Zoghbi W, Kronzon I, Mays JM, Pearlman AS, Schnittger I, et al. Echocardiography in emergency medicine: a policy statement by the American Society of Echocardiography and the American College of Cardiology. J Am Soc Echocardiogr 1999; 12:82–84.
17. Alexander JH, Peterson ED, Chen AY, Harding TM, Adams DB, Kisslo JA Jr. Feasibility of point-of-care echocardiography by internal medicine housestaff. Am Heart J 2004; 147:76–481.
18. Jones AE, Tayal VS, Kline JA. Focused training of emergency medicine residents in goal-directed echocardiography: a prospective study. Acad Emerg Med 2003; 10:1054–1058.
19. Benjamin E, Griffin K, Leibowitz AB, Manasia A, Oropello JM, Geffroy V, DelGiudice R, Hufanda J, Rosen S, Goldman M. Goal-directed transesophageal echocardiography performed by intensivists to assess left ventricular function: Comparison with pulmonary artery catheterization. J Cardiothorac Vasc Anesth 1998; 12:10–15.
20. Otto CM. Textbook of Clinical Echocardiography. 2d ed. Philadelphia, PA: W.B. Saunders Co., 2004.
21. Oh JK, Seward JN, Tajij JA. The Echo Manual. 2d ed. Philadelphia, PA: Lippincott Williams and Wilkins, 2000.
22. Feigenbaum H. Echocardiography. 6th ed. Philadelphia, PA: Lippincott Williams and Wilkins, 2005.
23. Weyman AE. Principles and Practice of Echocardiography. 1st ed. Philadelphia, PA: Lippincott Williams and Wilkins, 1993.
24. Otto CMPractice of Clinical Echocardiography. 2d ed. Philadelphia, PA: W.B. Saunders Co., 2002.
25. Weyman AE, Butler A, Subhiyah R, Appleton C, Geiser E, Goldstein SA, King ME, Kaul S, Labovitz A, Picard M, et al. Concept, development, administration and analysis of a certifying examination in echocardiography for physicians. J Am Soc Echocardiogr 2001; 14:158–168.
26. Pearson AC, Castello R, Labovitz AJ. Safety and utility of transesophageal echocardiography in the critically ill patient. Am Heart J 1990; 119:1083–1089.
27. Pavlides GS, Hauser AM, Stewart JR, O'Neill WW, Timmis GC. Contribution of transesophageal echocardiography to patient diagnosis and treatment: a prospective analysis. Am Heart J 1990; 120:910–914.
28. Foster E, Schiller NB. The role of transesophageal echocardiography in critical care: UCSF experience. J Am Soc Echocardiogr 1992; 5:368–374.
29. Hwang JJ, Shyu KG, Chen JJ, Tseng YZ, Kuan P, Lien WP. Usefulness of transesophageal echocardiography in the treatment of critically ill patients. Chest 1993; 104:861–866.
30. Vignon P, Mentec H, Terre S, Gastinne H, Gueret P, Lemaire F. Diagnostic accuracy and therapeutic impact of transthoracic and transesophageal echocardiography in the mechanically ventilated patients in the ICU. Chest 1994; 106:1820–1834.
31. Khoury AF, Afridi I, Quinones MA, Zoghbi WA. Transesophageal echocardiography in critically ill patients: feasibility, safety, and impact on management. Am Heart J 1994; 127:1363–1371.
32. Poelaert JI, Trouerbach J, De Buyzere M, Everaert J, Colardyn FA. Evaluation of transesophageal echocardiography as a diagnostic and therapeutic aid in a critical care setting. Chest 1995; 107:774–779.
33. Heidenreich PA, Stainback RF, Redberg RF, Schiller NB, Cohen NH, Foster E. Transesophageal echocardiography predicts mortality in critically ill patients with unexplained hypotension. J Am Coll Cardiol 1995; 26:152–158.

34. Alam M. Transesophageal echocardiography in critical care units: Henry Ford Hospital experience and review of the literature. Prog Cardiovasc Dis 1996; 38:315–328.

35. Slama MA, Novara A, Van de Putte P, Diebold B, Safavian A, Safar M, Ossart M, Fagon JY. Diagnostic and therapeutic implications of transesophageal echocardiography in medical ICU patients with unexplained shock, hypoxemia, or suspected endocarditis. Intensive Care Med 1996; 22:916–922.

36. Poelaert J, Schmidt C, Colardyn F. Transoesophageal echocardiography in the critically ill. Anaesthesia 1998; 53:55–68.

37. Colreavy FB, Donovan K, Lee KY, Weekes J. Transesophageal echocardiography in critically ill patients. Crit Care Med 2002; 30:989–996.

38. Liebson PR. Transesophageal echocardiography in critically ill patients: what is the intensivist's role? Crit Care Med 2002; 30:1165–1166.

39. Pruszcyk P, Torbicki A, Pacho R, Chlebus M, Kuch-Wocial A, Pruszynski B, Gurba H. Noninvasive diagnosis of suspected severe pulmonary embolism: transesophageal echocardiography vs spiral CT. Chest 1997; 112:722–728.

40. Vieillard-Baron A, Qanadli SD, Antakly Y, Fourme T, Loubieres Y, Jardin F, Dubourg O. Transesophageal echocardiography for the diagnosis of pulmonary embolism with acute cor pulmonale: a comparison with radiological procedures. Intensive Care Med 1998; 24:429–433.

41. Jardin F, Dubourg O, Bourdarias JP. Echocardiographic pattern of acute cor pulmonale. Chest 1997; 111:209–217.

42. Vieillard-Baron A, Prin S, Chergui K, Dubourg O, Jardin F. Echo-Doppler demonstration of acute cor pulmonale at the bedside in the medical intensive care unit. Am J Respir Crit Care Med 2002; 166:1310–1319.

43. Tsang TSM, Enriquez-Sarano M, Freeman WK, Barnes ME, Sinak LJ, Gersh BJ, Bailey KR, Seward JB. Consecutive 1127 therapeutic echocardiographically guided pericardiocenteses: clinical profile, practice patterns, and outcomes spanning 21 years. Mayo Clinic Proc 2002; 77:429–436.

44. Brown J. Use of echocardiography for hemodynamic monitoring. Crit Care Med 2002; 30:1361–1364.

45. Boussuges A, Blanc P, Molenat F, Burnet H, Habib G, Sainty JM. Evaluation of left ventricular filling pressure by transthoracic Doppler echocardiography in the intensive care unit. Crit Care Med 2002; 30:362–367.

46. Greim CA, Roewer N, Apfel C, Laux G, Schulte am Esch J. Relation of echocardiographic preload indices to stroke volume in critically ill patients with normal and low cardiac index. Intensive Care Med 1997; 23:411–416.

47. Leung JM, Levine EH. Left ventricular end-systolic cavity obliteration as an estimate of intraoperative hypovolemia. Anesthesiology 1994; 81:1102–1109.

48. Cheung AT, Savino JS, Weiss SJ, Aukburg SJ, Berlin JA. Echocardiographic and hemodynamic indexes of left ventricular preload in patients with normal and abnormal ventricular function. Anesthesiology 1994; 81:376–387.

49. Feissel M, Michard F, Mangin I, Ruyer O, Faller JP, Teboul JL. Respiratory changes in aortic blood velocity as an indicator of fluid responsiveness in ventilated patients with septic shock. Chest 2001; 119:867–873.

50. Vieillard-Baron A, Chergui K, Augarde R, Prin S, Page B, Beauchet A, Jardin F. Cyclic changes in arterial pulse during respiratory support revisited by Doppler echocardiography. Am J Respir Crit Care Med 2003; 168(6):671–676.

51. Cook CH, Praba AC, Beery PR, Martin LC. Transthoracic echocardiography is not cost-effective in critically ill surgical patients. J Trauma 2002; 52(2):280–284.

52. Lichtenstein D, Axler O. Intensive use of general ultrasound in the intensive care unit. Prospective study of 150 consecutive patients. Intensive Care Med 1993; 19:353–355.

53. Vieillard-Baron A, Prin S, Chergui K, Dubourg O, Jardin F. Hemodynamic instability in sepsis: bedside assessment by Doppler echocardiography. Am J Respir Crit Care Med 2003; 168:1270–1276.
54. Manasia AR, Nagaraj HM, Kodali RB, Croft LB, Oropello JM, Kohli-Seth R, Leibowitz AB, DelGiudice R, Hufanda JF, Benjamin E, Goldman ME. Feasibility and potential clinical utility of goal-directed transthoracic echocardiaography performed by noncardiologist intensivists using a small hand-carried device (Sono Heart) in critically ill patients. J Cardiothorac Vasc Anesth 2005; 19:155–159.

9

Documentation

Michael J. Simoff

Interventional Pulmonology and Bronchoscopy Services, Henry Ford Medical Center, Detroit, Michigan, U.S.A.

INTRODUCTION

Documentation is the collation, synopsizing, and coding of printed material for future reference. It is also described as the act of supplying documents, supporting references, or records (1). In the practice of medicine, very little can be gained, whether it is on a daily basis with the management of in- or out-patients or performing advanced research on gene expression, if the information we gain each day is not appropriately documented.

Outside of the research realm, much of medical documentation is geared towards the medical record. Proper documentation of the medical record is required to ensure that all pertinent facts, findings, and observations regarding a patient are recorded in a chronologic fashion: past medical and surgical history, examinations, test results, treatments, and outcomes. By organizing the information this way, the documented medical record makes possible communication between health care providers, augmenting the abilities of physicians and other support staff to provide and monitor patients' progress throughout their disease process (2).

Medical records should not only be used to communicate medical information, but should also be viewed as legal documents subject to review in their own right. Records should be logical, concise, and as precise as possible (3). Other important reasons for comprehensive documentation include: accurate and complete payment for services provided, utilization review and quality of care evaluations, and data collation for research and education (2). It is only through regulated and complete documentation by all health care providers that the medical record will remain a comprehensive source of information, thoughts, and data to maximize the provision of medical care.

Ultrasound (US) is an efficient and reliable tool for thoracic imaging. US can be used for the assessment of pleural effusions, pleural masses, chest wall pathology, pneumothorax, and cardiac function. In addition, US can be used as a guide to the performance of procedures including thoracentesis, biopsies, and vascular access to name a few (4) (5–9). With the advent of endobronchial ultrasound (EBUS) and further US-guided procedures, there will be a definite growth in US use by chest physicians. Sound practice patterns must be established with regard to performance and documentation early in the development of this clinical tool.

REPORTS

Communications theory states that the transfer of information from one message source to the next is most efficient when "fewer binary digits per character or per unit time" are used (3). Basically, the more concise and logically presented the reports are, the more accurate is the information conveyed to the reader. Reports can be made most efficient by presenting the most important findings first, highlighting them to the reader. Leaving this information until later may minimize the significance of a finding by burying it within a report.

Typically, report formats have a section describing the findings, often with some discussion, followed by the interpreter's impressions. In a certain respect, this puts the most important information last. When a format is developed for US reporting, its presentation must be taken into account. Most reports include six elements for completeness: (i) normal and normal variant findings, (ii) pathology and anatomy, (iii) descriptions of those findings including size, shape, location, and measurements, (iv) a subjective measure of certainty of a particular finding (i.e., probable vs. possible vs. cannot exclude), (v) details regarding changes in the finding as compared to previous studies, and (vi) suggestions for other imaging that might provide more information (3).

A US study often requires a technician to perform the experiment, as well as the physician reader/interpreter. With the advancement of more US-specific technologies, many of the thoracic procedures are now performed by the physicians without the help of technicians [EBUS, trans-esophageal echocardiograms (TEE), vascular access imaging, etc.]. As more individuals become involved in the process of performing and interpreting procedures, a more definitive structure needs to be established regarding the performance of tests, to maximize the quality of the testing and the subsequent interpretation. One such way to improve this process is the development of protocols for the performance of ultrasounds. The American Institute of Ultrasound in Medicine (AIUM) has created such protocols for US examination of:

- Abdomen or retroperitoneum
- Antepartum obstetrical
- Breast
- Extracranial cerebrovascular

- Female pelvis
- Infant brain
- Prostate and surrounding structures
- Scrotal
- Thyroid and parathyroid
- Vascular/Doppler

Each of these protocols includes the following sections: Equipment, Documentation, and Care of Equipment, as well as Guidelines for the performance of the ultrasound examination for the identified structure and surrounding tissue.

The equipment section includes recommendations for the type of transducers as well as the optimal frequencies for the performance of the particular study (e.g., a real-time, transrectal transducer should be used with frequencies of 5 MHz or higher). The Care of Equipment section highlights the necessity of proper sheaths for probes, cleaning and basic maintenance of the US equipment, and sterilization recommendations.

An often-neglected component in documentation is that of the equipment, and most particularly the general maintenance and routine cleaning and sterilization of the equipment used. For the purposes of infection control and quality management, records on each piece of equipment used for the life of that unit must be maintained. This practice will ensure that a standard, complete, and accurate system is used for maintaining all equipment.

Not only the records for the individual equipment, but also a comprehensive record for the procedure unit where they are performed should be maintained. Either a written format or a computer database can be considered for recording this type of information. A procedure unit record should be maintained by date, and should include: (i) patient identification data, (ii) names of operators/endoscopists and assistants including nurses/technicians, (iii) procedures performed, (iv) indications for procedures, (v) anatomic extent of examination or procedure, (vi) duration of the procedure, (vii) findings, (viii) identification of all biopsies or other sampling performed, (ix) any therapeutic interventions instituted during the procedure, (x) a report of any complications, including late complications that may arise, and (xi) any limitations of the examination. By maintaining such records, quality assurance reviews and projects can take place to ensure a high level of excellence in the procedure suite.

It is also recommended by the AIUM that a complete sonographic evaluation of the system to be scanned (breast, scrotal, etc.) be performed and recorded at the time of all studies. The complete system review, as recommended by the appropriate protocols, provides specific steps and image specifications required. The protocols also often provide the scanner with supporting illustrations to guide correct imaging and transducer placement. By following this type of protocol, complete scanning of the desired system is ensured. Currently, there are no such protocols for thoracic ultrasound or EBUS and it is debatable if full examinations should be performed when US is used for procedure guidance only.

PROTOCOLS

Protocols are standards by which scanning and documentation of findings should be reported. The universal use of scanning protocols will ensure that different physicians will be able to interpret the same study similarly. Specifically, if all studies were performed and then recorded with random sequences, it would be nearly impossible to interpret the information provided accurately on all occasions. If chefs around the world did not use recipes, then Alfredo sauce would not be Alfredo sauce wherever you might eat. It is a fact that some sauces are better than others depending on the chef, but the bottom line is that it is the same sauce. Some technicians and physicians will perform and/or interpret studies better than others, but the studies must be performed in such a manner that they are in essence the same.

As an example of the concept of protocols, the following is from the guidelines for the performance of US examination of the prostate, from the AIUM:

> The prostate should be imaged in its entirety in at least two orthogonal planes, sagittal and axial or sagittal and coronal, from the apex to the base of the gland. In particular, the peripheral zone should be thoroughly imaged. The gland should be evaluated for size, echogenicity, symmetry, and continuity of margins. The periprostatic fat and vessels should be evaluated for asymmetry and disruption in echogenicity (10).

This statement gives several very important guidelines to the person performing the study, including the salient planes of imaging as well as the details which should be examined. It is important to remember that many structures identified by US examination are recognized not by their sonographic image alone, but by their location. US images may be altered due to pathology within the organ being examined and therefore will not convey the expected image. Documented areas of interest must be imaged in a logical sequence to ensure proper and complete interpretation of the US examination.

STUDY DOCUMENTATION

Surveys are a portion of the examination, which allow the sonographer to get "the lay of the land" so to speak. Thorough and methodical surveys of the structures to be examined in at least two scanning planes prior to the performance of the actual examination is a recommended practice. This type of scout imaging will allow the sonographer to be prepared for any anatomic aberrancies and/or pathologic findings prior to the formal performance and recording of the examination.

Once the sonographer has performed the survey, formal image documentation must be completed. This is the study that must follow prescribed protocols. Important points to reiterate include that imaging must be performed in at least two scanning planes. Single-plane sonographic imaging of an abnormality does not provide the necessary information for confirmation of the finding. Complete documentation must include volume measurements of any abnormality identified with the appropriate images saved. This must be done at the time of the examination to ensure that the best possible images are saved for interpretation. Altering the gain in addition to varying the planes of view may help in the visualization of an abnormality. As in measurement, once the study is complete, if documentation regarding changes in the plane of scanning or modifications in gain used for viewing are not available to the reading physician, it may alter the interpretation of this study.

The video images produced at the time of the US examination will be used in the interpretation. Still images obtained at the time of the examination may be attached to the permanent medical record in addition to the interpretation of these images. Retention of the images produced, as part of the US examination, should be consistent both with the clinical need and with the relevant legal and local health care facility requirements. Image review may be important for comparison in future examinations, or in review of secondary findings otherwise not commented upon.

US examination has been part of the evaluation and management of obstetrical cases for a while. Both the American College of Obstetrics and Gynecology (ACOG) and AIUM produced standards and guidelines for performing obstetric US examinations, ACOG in 1988 (11) and AIUM in 1990 (12). Although the ACOG and AIUM publications were originally created as guidelines, they are now often referred to as the standard of care for the performance of such examinations. Smulian et al. (13) performed their study to determine the degree of documented compliance with ACOG and AIUM standardizations between an obstetrician's office and a radiologic facility (Table 1). Their findings demonstrated a poor compliance overall with the recommended documentation of US examinations. For second and third trimester US examinations, there was a 0% compliance with both ACOG and AIUM guidelines in the 129 studies reviewed, from both the obstetrician's offices and the radiology facilities.

Proper and complete documentation can be a time-consuming and tedious process; without it though, we would create a disorganized and in many ways useless record. There are no protocols for thoracic US examinations (except for echocardiography) currently. EBUS also has no standard protocol to dictate examination performance. A secondary difficulty with EBUS is that this test can be performed in only one plane for evaluation of an abnormality due to the environment in which the test is performed. For the advancement of thoracic ultrasonography, standards with appropriate protocols will need to be established for proper, reproducible, and clinically useful studies.

Table 1
Complete Compliance Rates of ACOG and AIUM Guidelines in First Vs. Second/Third Trimester Cases Reviewed

	Obstetrician's office		Radiologic facilities	
	ACOG (%)	AIUM (%)	ACOG (%)	AIUM (%)
First trimester reports (*n* = 46)	35	15	11.5	3.9
Second/third trimester reports (*n* = 129)	0	0	0	0

REPORT DOCUMENTATION

All endoscopic procedures should be documented in a complete and legible report. This report should be designed to be a part of the patient's medical record. To improve documentation of reports, a standardized approach for the reporting and recording of sonographic findings and abnormalities is important for an organized and easily usable report. The American Society for Gastrointestinal Endoscopy (ASGE) saw the necessity for a uniform approach to the performance and documentation of endoscopic studies. The ASGE created their original document, "Appropriate use of Gastrointestinal Endoscopy" (14) as a concensus statement. The goal of this document was to identify indications for procedure: in hopes of establishing local standards of endoscopic utilization. In 1997, the ASGE created the "Policy and Procedure Manual for Gastrointestinal Endoscopy: Guidelines for Training and Practice" (15). This document clearly outlines aspects for procedure reporting as well as the creation of endoscopic unit records, which was identified as a necessary aspect for the performance of the procedure. The development of similar guidelines for thoracic ultrasonography will need to be considered for the advancement of this technology.

An important issue regarding proper report documentation would be the use of verbiage correct to sonography. Those physicians in particular who are using US technology, yet are not trained as sonographers, must be cautious in the use of US-specific terminology. As an example, Table 2 includes a short list of terms used with sonographic appropriate definitions. Without a consistent use of specific terminology between technicians and physicians as well as between physicians and physicians, the information gained through US procedures will be of little benefit. As thoracic ultrasonography becomes a more common practice, specifics in the terminology must be chosen and decided upon for the standardization of this technology.

Furthermore, as abnormalities are identified, descriptions of the size, location, and composition of the findings must be clearly described. With regard to size, the abnormality should be scanned and measured in at least

Table 2 Sonographic Nomenclature	
Gray scale	Intensity of ultrasound signal brightness in terms of shades of gray
Echogenic	An echo-producing structure
Anechoic	An echo-free zone on the ultrasound image This appears as a black zone on the image, most commonly a fluid filled space
Hyperechoic	Descriptive term referring to an echo response brighter than the surrounding tissue and/or brighter than expected for the structure being evaluated
Hypoechoic/echopenic	Descriptive term referring to an echo response less bright than the surrounding tissue and/or less bright than expected for the structure being evaluated
Isoechoic/isosonic	Term suggesting that the echo-density of two structures is the same or nearly so
Heterogeneous	Term used to describe a nonuniform or uneven echopattern
Homogeneous	Term used to describe a uniform or even echopattern

Source: From Ref. 11.

two planes. This approach will allow the assessment of the size of the lesions in a more volumetric perspective. With further advancement in US technology, such as three-dimensional reconstruction, the recreation of pathologic findings will become more specific and in many ways easier. With the complete measurement of lesions, it is important to record in the report in what planes and/or at what locations the measurements were taken, to make it possible for another physician or technician to locate the identified lesion for follow-up comparison or to perform a procedure.

Precise representation of location of an abnormality is very important as part of the evaluation of a lesion. In EBUS for instance, description of the location within the airway that the US imaging was performed, using endobronchial landmarks, is a necessary component of the evaluation. Description of the anatomic structures surrounding the abnormality should also be used to improve relocating the identified lesion on subsequent evaluations or at the time of a procedure. It is also necessary to record the position the patient was in when the evaluation was performed. Pleural fluid evaluation, as an example, can be greatly altered by patient position (16).

Another important component of pathologic reporting is the description of the sonographic composition of the structure and/or abnormality identified. Using correct nomenclature (Table 2) as part of the description of the lesion is imperative. If high- and low-gain settings are varied to improve the characterization of an abnormality, this must also be recorded as part of the image documentation. Currently, sonographic images are not used to distinguish between malignant- and nonmalignant lesions, but research is ongoing in EBUS, to identify with high degrees of accuracy, the malignant and/or benign nature of a lesion by its sonographic characteristics (17).

THE REPORT

The documented report of a sonographic examination should include the date of the procedure as well as pertinent patient information: name, medical record number, and/or birth date. This section should also identify the relevant medical history and the indications for the procedure with the diagnosis (±ICD-9 code appropriate for the case).

The report of the procedure itself must include information regarding the equipment used for the procedure (transducers, frequency, and when appropriate endoscopic system). The names of the endoscopist, assistants, and support staff (nurses and/or assistants) must all be recorded as part of the documentation for the examination.

The findings of the examination should be comprehensively documented as reviewed above. The anatomic extent of the examination in addition to the pathologic or abnormal findings must be recorded. If there were limitations to the examination, this would be appropriately reported here. On occasions in which a procedure is performed in conjunction with the examination, records of the complete procedure should be included: anesthesia, site of procedure, samples acquired, and complications. Comparison to previous examinations, when applicable, should also be included in the final report (18).

SUMMARY

Complete documentation of all sonographic procedures is essential for high-quality patient care. A record must be created which includes pertinent imaging of both normal and abnormal findings, complete interpretation of the results, and the supporting information to have a comprehensive report. Documentation is an important form of communication between health care providers. Without clear, concise, and accurate records, performing the test itself will be of no benefit. Thoracic ultrasonography is an emerging field in medicine; establishing guidelines for the test and the documentation of the reports now will help it grow.

REFERENCES

1. The American Heritage Dictionary of the English Language. 3rd ed. Boston: Houghton Mifflin Company, 1996.
2. American Institute of Ultrasound in Medicine. 1997 Documentation Guidelines for Evaluation and Management Services. http://www.aium.org, 2003.
3. Beall DP. Radiology Sourcebook. Totowa: Humana Press, 2002:101–107.
4. Armstrong P, Wilson AG, Dee P, Hansell DM. Year Book. 2d ed. St. Louis: Mosby Inc., 1995.
5. Fraser RS, Pare PD, Colman N, Muller NL. Diagnosis of diseases of the chest. Vol. 1. 4th ed. Philadelphia: WB Saunders Company, 1999.
6. Rozycki GS, Pennington SD, Feliciano DV. Surgeon-performed ultrasound in the critical care setting: its use as an extension of the physical examination to detect pleural effusion. J Trauma 2001; 50:636–642.
7. Dulchavsky SA, Schwarz KL, Kirkpatrick AW, Billica RD, Williams DR, Diebel LN, Campbell MR, Sargysan AE, Hamilton DR. Prospective evaluation of thoracic ultrasound in the detection of pneumothorax. J Trauma 2001; 50:201–205.
8. Dulchavsky SA, Hamilton DR, Diebel LN, Sargysan AE, Billica RD, Williams DR. Thoracic ultrasound diagnosis of pneumothorax. J Trauma 1999; 47:970–971.
9. Brant WE. The Thorax. In: Rumack CM, Wilson SR, Charboneau JW, eds. Diagnostic Ultrasound. St Louis: Mosby-Year Book, 1991:413–428.
10. AIUM Guidelines for performance of the ultrasound examination of the prostate (and surrounding structures). In: Tempkin BB, ed. Ultrasound Scanning. 2d ed. Philadelphia: WB Saunders Company, 1999:463–465.
11. Hobbins J. Ultrasound in pregnancy. American College of Obstetricians and Gynecologists Technical Bulletin No. 116. Washington DC, 1988.
12. American Institute of Ultrasound in Medicine. Standards and Guidelines for Performance of the Antepartum Obstetrical Examination. 1990.
13. Smulian JC, Vintzileos AM, Rodis JF, Campbell WA. Community-based obstetrical ultrasound reports: documentation of compliance with suggested minimum standards. J Clin Ultrasound 1996; 24:123–127.
14. American Society for Gastrointestinal Endoscopy. Appropriate use of gastrointestinal endoscopy. A consensus statement from the American Society for Gastrointestinal Endoscopy, Manchester, MA, 1986.
15. The American Society for Gastrointestinal Endoscopy. Guidelines for training and practice. Policy and procedure manual for gastrointestinal endoscopy. May 1997.
16. General principles. In: Tempkin BB, ed. Ultrasound Scanning. 2d ed. Philadelphia: WB Saunders Company, 1999:1–18.
17. Pathology scanning protocol. In: Tempkin BB, ed. Ultrasound Scanning. 2d ed. Philadelphia: WB Saunders Company, 1999:19–22.
18. AIUM standard for documentation of an ultrasound examination. American Institute of Ultrasound in Medicine, 2002.

10

Ultrasound: Future Directions

Christopher J. Harvey
Imaging Sciences Department, Imperial College, Hammersmith Hospital, London, U.K.

Martin J. K. Blomley
Imaging Sciences Department, Imperial College, Hammersmith Hospital, London, U.K.

David O. Cosgrove
Imaging Sciences Department, Imperial College, Hammersmith Hospital, London, U.K.

INTRODUCTION

In just three decades, diagnostic ultrasound (US) machines have progressed from cumbersome, expensive B-mode gantry systems that produced coarse, static, and bistable images to hand-held devices capable of high resolution, real time, gray-scale, and Doppler imaging. Modern US machines are fully digital, which not only improves the signal-to-noise ratio of the returning echoes but also has a huge potential for improving the performance of scanners with respect to beam formation, signal processing, image display, and archiving (1). US may also be used to measure the elastic and dynamic properties of tissues. Technological advances have resulted in novel imaging modes such as those which exploit the nonlinear behavior of tissue and microbubble contrast agents. Microbubbles are safe and effective vascular echo-enhancers which have extended the versatility of US and allow microcirculation to be imaged, besides providing functional data. They also have potential as tissue-specific and targeted therapeutic agents. US has recently moved into therapeutic applications with high intensity focused ultrasound (HIFU) and microbubble-assisted delivery of drugs and genes showing great promise. It is a testament to the importance of US that over 25% of all imaging studies worldwide are US examinations. This chapter describes recent advances in US and contrast media and likely future developments.

A

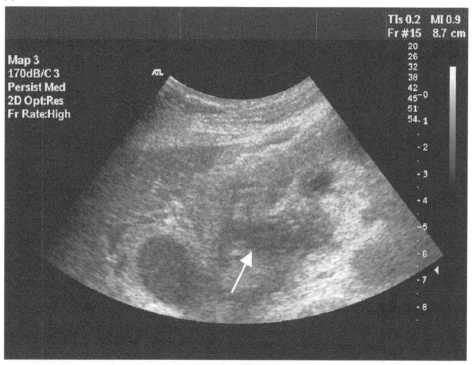

B

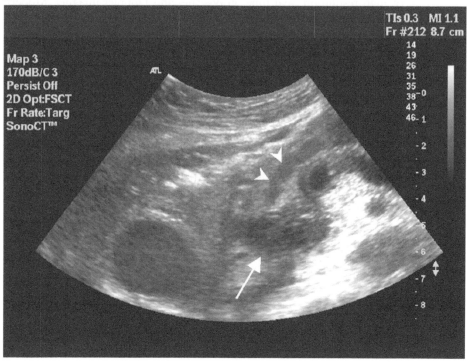

COMPONENTS OF A REAL-TIME B-MODE ULTRASOUND SYSTEM

Real-time B-mode is most commonly used in clinical scanning and so it is important to outline the mechanisms by which such images are produced. Each image is formed line by line based on information from the transducer which transmits and receives the US signals. The US echoes are converted by the transducer into electrical radiofrequency (RF) signals which undergo amplification [influenced by the time gain compensation (TGC)]. In the scanner, the digitizer converts these analogue signals into RF digital signals and the amplitude, or envelope, of these signals is detected. This information is then read into the image memory (scan convertor) where it is converted into a format appropriate for visual display. The image data is usually manipulated by postprocessing, logarithmic compression, and interpolation between scan lines. Developments at each stage of this pathway enhance the final image and these will be described.

Developments in Transducer Materials and Construction

The extensive selection of transducers available is a testament to the diversity of US applications and indeed some of the most significant advances in image quality and applications follow from innovations in transducer technology (2). Broadband technology has facilitated the development of nonlinear and harmonic imaging and has improved contrast and spatial resolution (3). Future transducer developments will depend on array configurations, transducer materials, and construction with the promise of higher frequency probes, higher element densities, innovative geometries, advances in beam-forming, and improved ferroelectrics (4).

From the surface, a typical transducer comprises (i) a protective layer, (ii) a focusing lens, (iii) matching layers, (iv) an active ferro- or piezoelectric material (with electrodes and connections), and (v) a backing block. The increase in bandwidth is due to the advances made by manufacturers in producing multiple matching layers thereby maximizing the electromechanical coupling coefficient (a measure of the efficiency of conversion of sound to electrical energy). The ferroelectric material used is paramount in the performance of the transducer. New piezoelectric materials, known as ferroelectric relaxors, are currently under evaluation (5). They are much more efficient in the conversion of electrical energy to sound energy, with an acoustic impedance better matched to tissue than to traditional piezoelectric materials.

Figure 1
Axial section of the pancreas in a 78-year-old lady presenting with obstructive jaundice: (**A**) The B-mode image shows an ill-defined lesion in the pancreatic head (*arrow*). (**B**) Compound imaging (SonoCT; Philips, Bothell, WA, U.S.) clearly defines a pancreatic head mass (*arrow*) with associated obstruction of the pancreatic duct (*arrowheads*). *Source*: From Ref. 75.

A

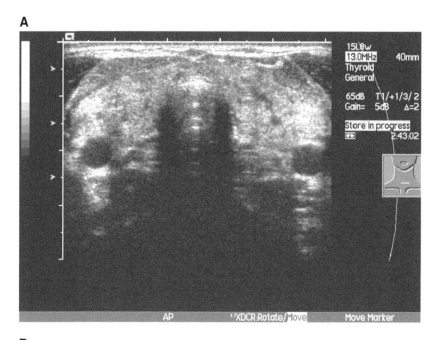

B

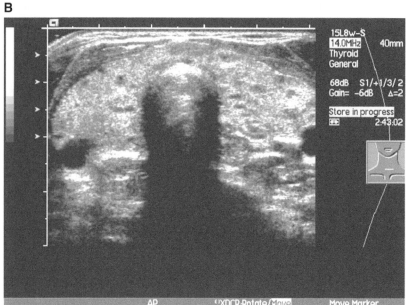

Figure 2
Axial section of the thyroid in a case of multinodular goitre: (**A**) The B-mode image (13 MHz) shows multiple ill-defined thyroid nodules. (**B**) In coded excitation mode (Chirp), the higher frequencies (14 MHz) can be utilized to improve spatial and contrast resolution down to greater depths so that the multinodular pattern is clearly demonstrated. *Source*: From Ref. 75.

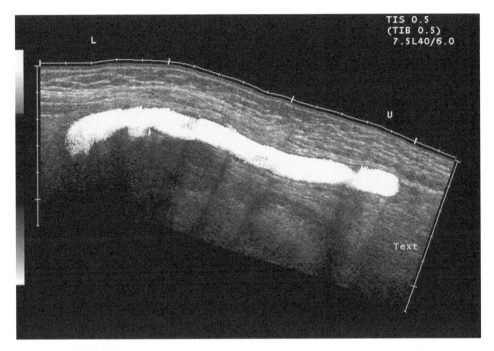

Figure 3
An extended field of view power Doppler image (Cscape, Siemens, Germany)
showing a recanalized paraumbilical vein in a patient with portal hypertension.
Abbreviations: L, liver; U, umbilicus. *Source*: From Ref. 75.

Digital Ultrasonic Imaging

Digital technology has revolutionized all stages of Ultrasonography
systems (6). One of the most important advances is the use of

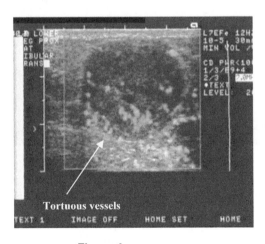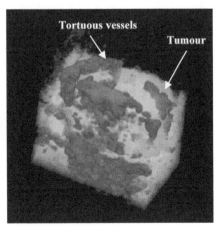

Figure 4
Tortuous vessels in a neurilemmoma, appreciated in both 2D and 3D. *Source*:
Courtesy of Dr. V. Jayaram. From Ref. 75.

A

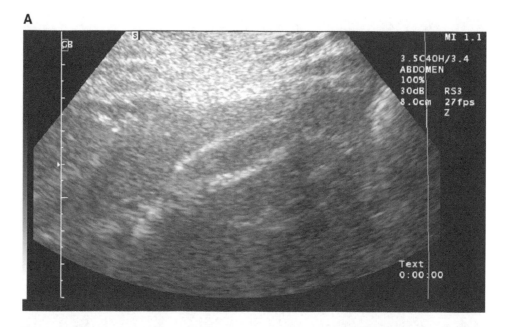

B

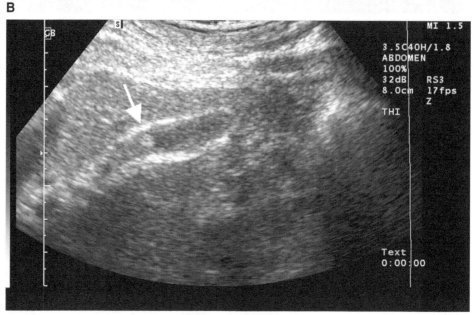

Figure 5
Section through the gallbladder of a 56-year-old lady presenting with abdominal pain: (**A**) The B-mode image suggests an ill-defined echogenic lesion in the gallbladder which is difficult to characterize further. (**B**) Scanning in THI (Siemens, Germany), an echogenic 3 mm gallbladder polyp is clearly demonstrated (*arrow*). *Abbreviations*: THI, Tissue harmonic imaging. *Source*: From Ref. 75.

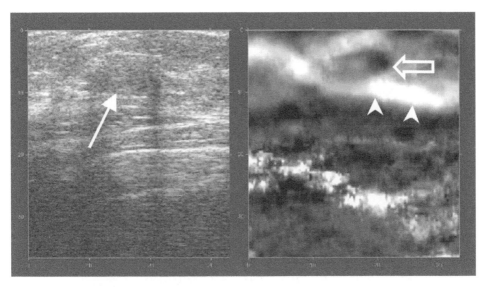

Figure 6
On the left, a conventional B-mode breast image shows a well-circumscribed, echo-poor fibroadenoma (*arrow*). On the right, an elastogram of the same lesion shows the hard outer rim of tissue (*open arrow*) in black with the softer central tissue in gray-white. The white line (*arrowheads*) is the chest wall. *Source:* Courtesy of Dr. F. Fuechsel. From Ref. 75.

Application-Specific Integrated Circuits (ASICs) whereby one super chip can replace several boards of electronics. ASICs mean that circuit complexity, speed, and reliability can be increased whilst reducing relative cost, power consumption, and size. Thus we have seen the evolution of small portable scanners with high resolution gray scale, power and pulsed wave Doppler, tissue harmonic imaging, and image/cine memory.

Digital beam forming has allowed the development of time-saving techniques which may be used to improve image quality, the size of the field of view, or the frame rate.

Digital control of the transducer array is used to steer the US beam and allows dynamic changes in both focusing and aperture to be made while receiving US echoes. This provides higher spatial resolution and, by reducing artifacts, improves image contrast.

Image/Signal Processing

A number of ingenious techniques have been developed by manufacturers to optimize US images by manipulating the RF digital signal, thus improving diagnostic efficiency and reducing the operator-dependent nature of US. Spatial compounding is a technique which uses electronic beam steering of the transducer array to acquire overlapping scans (varying 3–9 frames) of an object from different angles. The scan lines are then averaged to produce a real-time compound image of improved quality

A

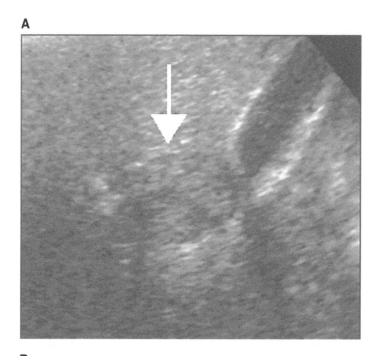

B

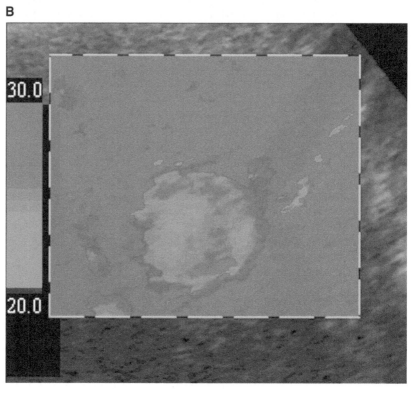

(better contrast resolution compared with the conventional B-mode image) because of reduction in speckle (Fig. 1). Compound imaging has found applications in many areas including imaging of the abdomen, peripheral vasculature, breast, and musculoskeletal system (7).

Coded excitation is a technique that has been developed from technology used in radar. The basis of this technology is that the transmitted pulse is digitally encoded and the frequency response of the receiver is optimized according to the application and target depth. For example, the transmitted pulse can be modified by varying the frequency or amplitude. This "code" can be looked for in the returning echoes thereby allowing weak echoes to be distinguished from background noise. The advantages are that higher frequencies improve spatial and contrast resolution to greater depths (Fig. 2). In addition, the technique has been modified to image flowing blood in B-mode without contrast agents (B-flow, GE Medical Systems and Dynaflow, Toshiba Medical Systems, Japan).

Automatic gain compensation modes set the correct gain in 2D at any point across the image at the press of a button. This is achieved by the processor, analyzing the distribution of gray levels in each part of the image and adjusting the gray level of each pixel to optimize local contrast. These modes may help reduce the operator dependence of US. Automatic optimization systems are also available for power and spectral Doppler.

Extended Field of View Ultrasound

When US was introduced into clinical practice in the 1970s, articulated arm scanners were used to produce extended field of view US (EFOV) images but this was given up when real-time US was developed. However, technological advances in computing mean that we can now produce high resolution EFOV images in gray scale or Doppler (Fig. 3). EFOV imaging can be performed on superficial structures using linear array transducers or in abdominal/pelvic studies with a curvilinear probe (8). The value of this technique is the fact that lesions and their anatomical relationships can easily be depicted for clinicians and radiologists; it is an excellent teaching aid, which allows measurements of large structures to be taken and serves as a useful record for follow-up. EFOV is most useful for superficial structures, such as the neck, scrotum, musculoskeletal system, and breast (9).

Figure 7
Functional image of the right lobe of liver in a 58-year-old man with metastatic insulinoma: (**A**) B-mode image showing a metastasis (*arrow*). (**B**) A functional overlay has been superimposed on the image depicting arrival time of microbubbles after a bolus injection (range 20–30 sec). Note the early arrival time (< 25 sec) of contrast agent in the metastasis compared to the adjacent parenchyma. *Source*: From Ref. 33.

A

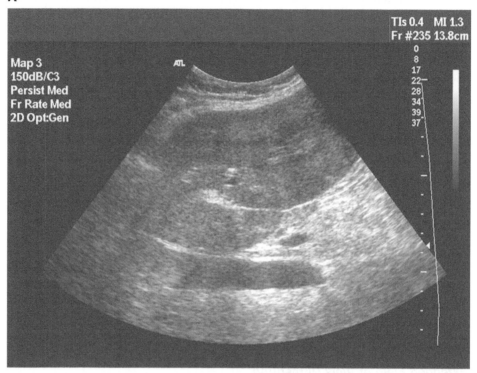

B

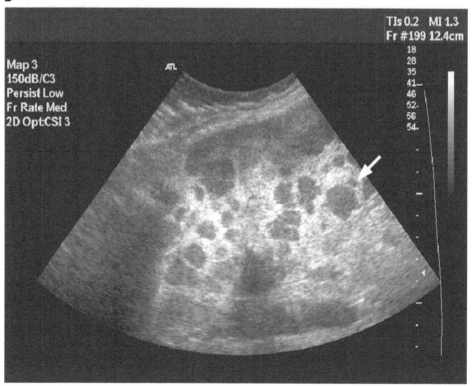

Three-Dimensional (3D) Ultrasound

Until relatively recently, US lagged behind both computerized tomography (CT) and magnetic resonance (MR) in 3D imaging (10,11). 3D US is based on reconstruction algorithms and is therefore dependent on high quality 2D data which have been limited by problems, such as speckle, grating lobe, clutter, and other artifacts. Recent developments in harmonic imaging, nonlinear signal processing, and 2D matrix array transducers have reduced these problems. Advances in computing power have resulted in the recent production of a real-time 3D scanner (so-called 4D US imaging) (Voluson® 730, Kretztechnik AG, Zipf, Austria). Volume data can be displayed either as a series of multiplanar reformats (MPR) or as a rendered image allowing optimal appreciation of the relative position of structures, including flowing blood, within that volume. Clinical applications are diverse and include obstetrics, intravascular intervention, echocardiography, and breast/small parts and tumor vascularity (Fig. 4). 3D US has been shown to be a useful supplement to 2D US in the assessment of the fetal face (12) and skeleton and in volume measurements in obstretics and oncology. In the interventional setting, 3D US (13) is used to guide radioactive seed implants in the prostate, insertion of transjugular intrahepatic portocaval shunts, and breast biopsy, while a stereotactic system has been developed for needle delivery using electromagnetic position sensors. 4D US has already found applications in echocardiography and in needle guidance systems.

New Imaging Modes

Tissue harmonic imaging (THI) is a gray-scale imaging technique that uses information from harmonic signals generated by the nonlinear propagation of a sound wave as it passes through the tissue (14,15). Nonlinear transmission occurs because sound travels faster through compressed tissue than through relaxed tissue and this results in distortion of the incident wave with production of higher frequency components which are multiples (harmonics) of the insonating fundamental frequency (16). Whilst conventional US transmits and receives at the same frequency, THI uses low transmit frequency and the second harmonic signal to form the image by separating it from the fundamental echoes using filters. Harmonic signals are generated within the tissue in the center of the US beam (where the tissue experiences the higher acoustic intensities

---

Figure 8
Longitudinal section of the left lobe of liver in a 74-year-old man with carcinoma of the colon: (**A**) Conventional B-mode shows a heterogenous liver echotexture but no definite focal lesions. (**B**) Interrogation of the same area in PIM (Philips, Bothell, WA, U.S.) following Levovist reveals multiple metastases, some as small as 3 mm (*arrow*). Note the characteristic bright halo around the metastases. *Abbreviation*: PIM, pulse inversion mode. *Source*: From Ref. 55.

A

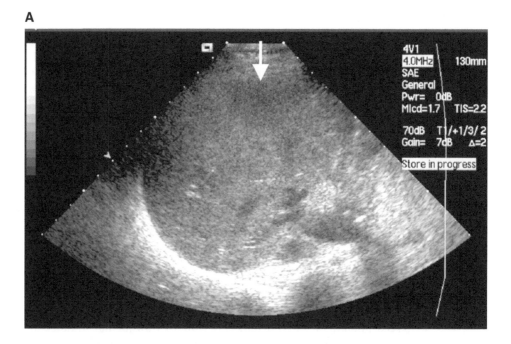

B

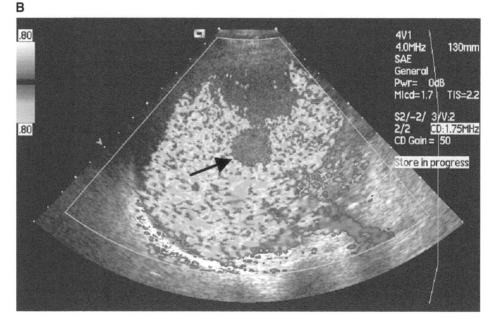

Figure 9
Section through the right lobe of liver in a 76-year-old man with pancreatic carcinoma: (**A**) The baseline B-mode image shows a subtle metastasis (*arrow*). (**B**) Imaging in stimulated acoustic emission (SAE) mode three minutes after Levovist not only improves the conspicuity of the metastasis but also reveals a further metastasis (*arrow*) which cannot be seen in B-mode. *Source*: From Ref. 75.

A

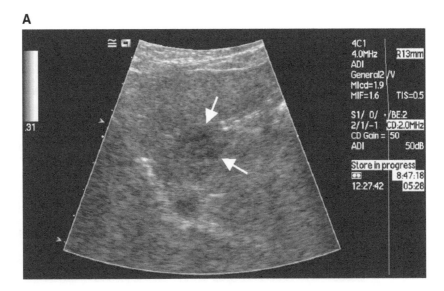

B

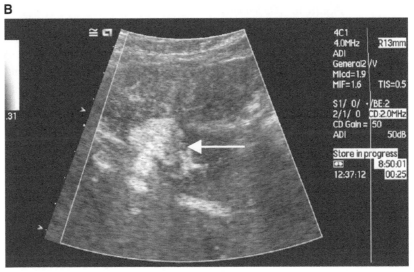

Figure 10
This 34-year-old man presented with abdominal pain: (**A**) The B-mode image shows an echo-poor lesion in the left lobe of the liver (*arrows*). (**B**) 25 seconds after a bolus injection of Levovist, the vascular phase was imaged in agent detection imaging mode (ADI; Siemens, CA, U.S.A.) and shows the lesion to be hypervascular (*arrow*) suggesting FNH. (**C**) Imaging in the liver-specific phase of Levovist (five minutes after injection) in ADI mode shows signal within the lesion (*arrows*), equal to adjacent liver parenchyma, which supports the diagnosis of FNH which was subsequently confirmed. *Abbreviations*: FNH, focal nodular hyperpalsia. *Source*: From Ref. 75.

C

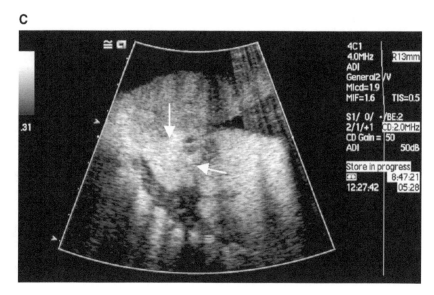

Figure 10 (Continued)

necessary for nonlinear behavior). The result is that the beam profile is improved because the weaker nonharmonic signals from multiple reflections at the body wall (especially in the obese) and side-lobes do not contribute to the final harmonic image. Therefore THI improves the signal-to-noise ratio and so the contrast resolution.

This technique is particularly well suited for imaging the "technically difficult" obese patient, the retroperitoneum, and pelvic pathology (17,18). Its value has been demonstrated in hepatic sonography where it provides extra information which alters management and reveals lesions not seen on conventional B-mode even in cirrhotic patients (19–21). Harmonic imaging increases diagnostic confidence in differentiating cystic from solid hepatic lesions, improves detection of stones in the gallbladder and biliary tree, improves pancreatic definition, and allows distinction of simple cysts from complex renal cysts. It is also very important in echocardiography (Fig. 5) (17,18).

Alternative Ultrasonic Imaging Methods

A number of ultrasonic imaging methods that are currently being evaluated utilize physical behaviors of tissue alternative to those used in B-mode scanning (i.e., bulk modulus) to produce their image.

Elastography

The stiffness (Young's modulus) of tissue tends to alter (usually increase) with pathology and can be imaged by measuring the tissue's distortion (strain) under an applied stress (e.g., compression via the transducer). Using this technique, known as elasticity imaging, or elastography, the difference between pathological tissue and surrounding normal tissue

A

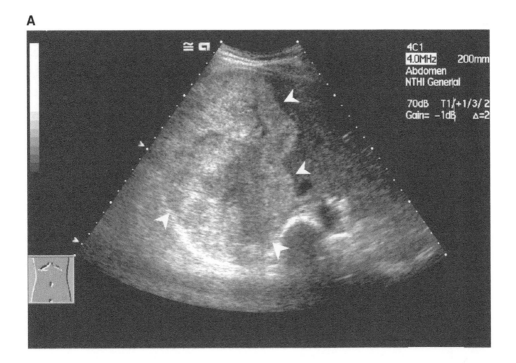

B

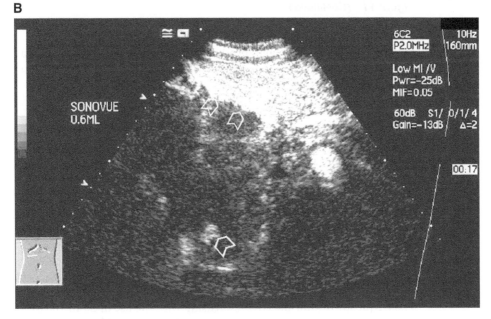

Figure 11
Hemangioma in a 47-year-old lady: (**A**) The baseline US shows a large heterogeneous liver lesion (*arrowheads*). (**B**) Following a bolus injection of Sonovue
(Bracco, Italy) the vascular phase was imaged using the novel real-time nondestructive contrast pulse sequence mode (CPS; Siemens, CA, U.S.). Characteristic
peripheral globular enhancement (*arrows*) is present. (**C**) After several minutes
continuous imaging centripedal lesion filling-in (*arrows*) is seen, strongly sugges-
tive of a hemangioma. *Abbreviation*: US, ultrasonography. *Source*: From Ref. 75.

C

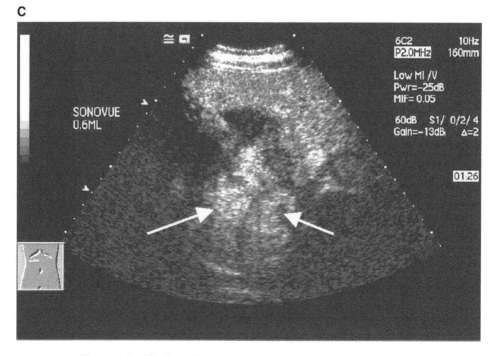

Figure 11   *(Continued)*

can be quantified. The images produced have very high contrast and may significantly improve lesion detection within the breast, prostate, blood vessels, and liver (Fig. 6) (22,23).

Vibro-Acoustography

This is another method for imaging tissue elasticity and is achieved by focusing two US beams with slightly different frequencies on an object of interest. The resulting interference causes the object to vibrate at a low frequency which is detected by a microphone (hydrophone). By scanning the two focused beams across the object, an image is built up. This technique appears to be particularly adept at delineating calcium deposits within tissues, such as breast microcalcifications (24).

Acoustic Microscopy

The frequency of transducers is increasing with the use of 30 to 100 MHz probes a realistic proposition early in the 21st century. These transducers rely on single element mechanical devices and are based on the ferroelectric polymer polyvinylidene fluoride (PVDF), which has a high bandwidth (>100%) but relatively poor sensitivity. Applications in ophthalmology and acoustic microscopy have been developed. US is poised to play an important role in the diagnosis and treatment of ocular

A

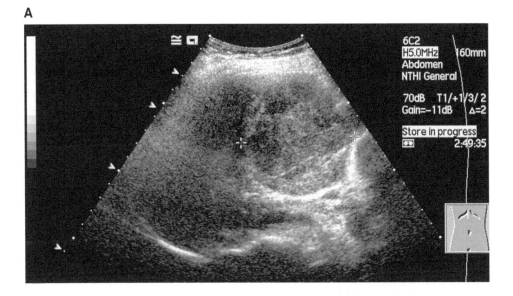

B

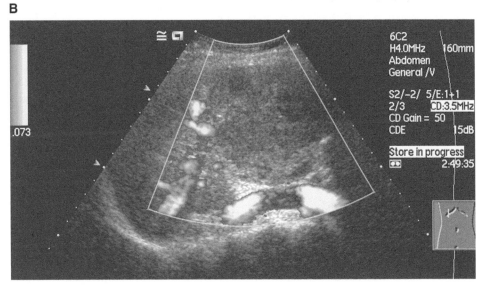

Figure 12
Follow-up US in a 46-year-old lady who had undergone chemoembolization of
an HCC: (**A**) The baseline US shows an HCC with areas of necrosis. (**B**) Power
Doppler interrogation shows no evidence of tumor recurrence. (**C**) Following a
bolus injection of the microbubble Sonovue (Bracco, Italy) the vascular phase
was imaged using contrast coherent imaging mode (CCI; Siemens, CA, U.S.)
and shows an avidly enhancing peripheral lesion (*arrow*) which was confirmed
to be a recurrent HCC. *Abbreviations*: HCC, hepatocellular carcinoma; US,
ultrasonography. *Source*: From Ref. 75.

C

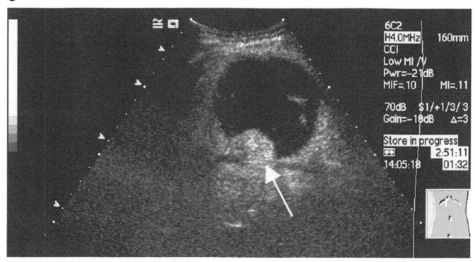

Figure 12 *(Continued)*

diseases ranging from tumors, through retinal and vitreous conditions (seen in diabetes and trauma) to anterior chamber pathologies such as glaucoma. Acoustic microscopy utilizes a number of acoustic tissue characteristics such as attenuation and impedance to produce an image (25). The technique has been applied to dermatological conditions, stomach tumors, and the kidney (26–28). Acoustic microscopy is not yet a widespread diagnostic tool but it should soon be possible to insert an ultrahigh frequency microtransducer, via a fine bore needle, into tissue and obtain in situ histology (25).

Endoluminal Ultrasound

The miniaturization of transducers has allowed interrogation of a wide variety of lumina (29). There are now nanoprobes which can be inserted through a 21 gauge needle and catheters. These have found application in the gastrointestinal tract, biliary system, urogenital tract, and tracheobronchial tree allowing difficult-to-access lesions to be fully characterized and biopsed. In the future, therapy may be administered via this route.

Intravascular US (IVUS), in which the vessel wall is displayed at 10 to 30 MHz, has been applied to the coronary and carotid arteries allowing plaque characterization and calculation of blood flow and shear wall stresses (30). IVUS may also be used to guide and monitor angioplasty.

Microbubble Contrast Agents

US, unlike all other imaging modalities, lacked effective contrast agents until comparatively recently. This was rectified with the introduction of

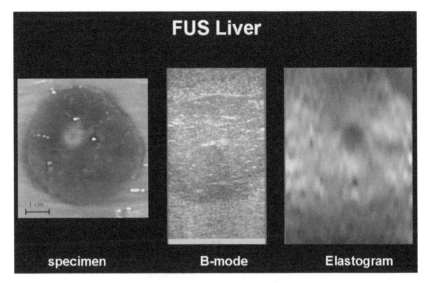

Figure 13
(*left*) Cross-section of a lesion produced by an HIFU beam in liver ex vivo.
(*middle*) B-mode image in which the lesion is ill-defined. (*right*) Elastogram in
which the lesion is clearly visualized. *Abbreviation:* HIFU, high intensity focused
ultrasound. *Source*: Courtesy of Dr. J. Bamber and Dr. M. Doyley. From Ref. 75.

microbubbles in the 1990s, which have revolutionized clinical and
research applications in this field (31–33). Microbubbles are < 10 μm
in diameter, so they can cross capillary beds, and are safe, effective echo
enhancers. When administered intravenously, microbubbles remain
within the vascular compartment, though recently some agents have been
shown to exhibit a hepatosplenic, tissue-specific phase (Table 1). To be
effective as clinical tools, microbubbles must survive passage through
the cardiopulmonary circulation to produce useful systemic enhancement. An ingenious range of methods are employed to achieve stability
and provide a clinically useful enhancement period. Microbubbles consist
of a gas (air or a perfluorocarbon) which is stabilized by a shell (dena-
tured albumin, phospholipid, surfactant, or cyanoacrylate) (Table 1).
Microbubbles cause a marked augmentation in the US signal for several
minutes after an intravenous bolus or 15 to 20 minutes after an infusion
with enhancement, in gray scale and Doppler signals of up to 25 dB
(> 300-fold increase).

The interactions of microbubbles with a US beam are complex
(34,35). Since a microbubble is more compressible than soft tissue, when
it is exposed to an oscillating acoustic signal, alternate expansion and
contraction occurs. At low acoustic power (< 100 KPa), these oscillations
are equal and symmetrical (linear behavior) and the frequency of the scattered signal is unaltered. As the acoustic power increases (100 KPa to
1 MPa), microbubbles resonate (nonlinear behavior) and behave like a

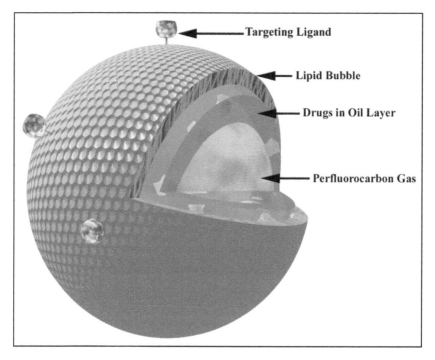

Figure 14
Schematic diagram of a microbubble manufactured for drug delivery. The interior of a microbubble may be loaded with drugs and gas. A stabilizing material, in this case a lipid, surrounds the perfluorocarbon gas. Drugs may be incorporated by themselves or, if insoluble, in an oil layer. Protein ligands on the microbubble surface may be targeted to a specific tissue. *Source*: From Ref. 76.

musical instrument emitting harmonic signals at multiples (or fractions) of the insonating frequency. Some of these nonlinear signals are microbubble-specific and may be regarded as a signature or fingerprint unique to that agent. Still higher powers (although within accepted limits for diagnostic imaging) disrupt the microbubbles, and this may be imaged with a number of bubble-specific modes which allow differentiation of contrast signal from background tissue.

Harmonic Imaging

Harmonics may be used to image US contrast agents by tuning the receiver to listen to a band of frequencies centered on a harmonic signal (usually the second harmonic $2f_0$, where f_0 is the center frequency of the transmitted pulse) so that the contrast signal is separately resolved from the background tissue (16). This allows the microcirculation to be imaged and flow in vessels down to 100 μm in diameter to be demonstrated, permitting characterization of tumor vascularity (36). Three-dimensional displays can be constructed to demonstrate vascular

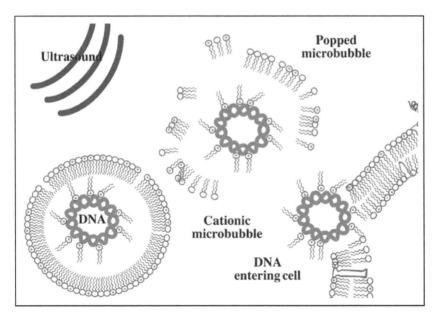

Figure 15
Gene delivery using microbubbles and US. US waves burst the gas-filled, gene-laden microbubbles and also cause sonoporation (transient nonlethal cell membrane perforation) which allows the genetic material to enter the target cells. *Abbreviation:* US, ultrasound. *Source:* From Ref. 76.

anatomy. This is a field with great potential, especially with the recent interest in monitoring the response of cancers to angiogenesis inhibitors. Harmonic imaging can be used to image the transient signals produced when microbubbles are disrupted at higher acoustic powers, and this is important for those agents that have a stationary tissue-specific phase, as discussed below.

Clinical Applications

Nonvascular uses include sonosalpingography in which fallopian tube patency is demonstrated by instilling Echovist into the uterine cavity and noting its passage along the tubes (37), and in the detection of vesico-ureteric reflux when Levovist is introduced into the bladder and the renal pelves and ureters are studied (38). Both of these techniques have the advantage of avoiding ionizing radiation and their sensitivity and specificity is comparable with those of conventional radiographic studies.

The most important routine clinical applications have been in the rescue or improvement of Doppler studies that would otherwise fail because of weak signals attenuated by overlying tissues (Table 2) (31–33,39).

Microbubbles have important applications in echocardiography (40). They are licenced for ventricular enhancement, and for delineation

Table 1
Classification of Ultrasound Microbubbles

Microbubble	Gas	Stabilization	Company
First generation vascular			
Agitated saline	Air	None	N/A
Echovist[a]	Air	None	Schering
Second generation vascular			
Levovist (SHU 508A)[a]	Air	Palmitic acid	Schering
Albunex[b]	Air	Sonicated albumin	Tyco
Third generation vascular			
Optison[a] (FS069)	Perfluoropropane	Sonicated albumin	Tyco
Echogen (QW3600)	Dodecafluoropentane	Liquid droplet, surfactant	Sonus
QW7437	Perfluorocarbon	Liquid droplet, surfactant	Sonus
Sonovue (BR1)[a]	Sulfur hexafluoride	Phospholipids	Bracco
Definity, (DMP115)	Perfluoropropane	Phospholipids	Bristol Meyer Squibb
PESDA	Perfluorobutane	Sonicated albumin	University of Nebraska
Quantison	Air	Dried albumin	Andaris Ltd
Imagent (AFO150)	Perfluorohexane	Surfactants	Schering
Liver specific agents			
Levovist (SHU 508A)	Air	Palmitic acid	Schering
Sonavist (SHU 563A)	Air	Cyanoacrylate	Schering
Sonazoid™ (NC100100)	Perfluorocarbon	Not public information	Amersham

[a]Licensed for clinical use.
[b]No longer commercially available.

of endocardial borders allowing improved detection of wall motion abnormalities as well as for converting nondiagnostic echocardiograms to diagnosticforms. The administration of contrast has been shown to enable more accurate measurement of left ventricular volume and ejection fraction, diagnosis and grading of valvular disease, thrombus detection, aortic dissection, detection of complications of myocardial infarction, such as ventricular rupture, and aneurysm formation and to improve the assessment of systolic function compared to B-mode imaging. In stress echocardiography, contrast agents increase the number of interpretable segments, especially in the endocardium, which allows accurate assessment of global and regional left ventricular function (41). At the myocardial level, contrast agents can be used to diagnose infarction and assess viability. Coronary artery stenoses can be localized and their severity quantified using intermittent harmonic imaging. Coronary flow rate (a measure of perfusion) may be calculated using bubble destruction and reperfusion methods, as discussed below (42). The assessment of myocardial perfusion is still experimental but with advances in US technology and contrast agents, the noninvasive echocardiographic diagnosis of both global and regional cardiac structure, function, and perfusion is on the horizon.

Novel Applications of Microbubbles

Quantitation and Functional Studies

Quantitation can be divided into "passive" and "active" methods. In the passive approach, the passage of a contrast bolus is recorded with minimal microbubble disruption; so, low insonating energies are employed. With active approaches, microbubbles are deliberately destroyed so that replenishment of a tissue bed can be measured while disruption of liver-specific agents produces strong transient enhancement when imaged in some nonlinear modes such as phase inversion mode.

Following a bolus injection of microbubbles, their passage through a tissue of interest such as a tumor or organ can be quantified to generate transit time curves, as with nuclear medicine, CT, and MR (43); from these, functional information can be derived to yield indices, such as bolus arrival time, time to peak intensity, area under the curve, and wash in/wash out characteristics.

An important application is the study of hepatic vascular transit times after a peripheral bolus injection of a microbubble, whilst interrogating a hepatic vein with spectral Doppler. Early arrival of contrast bolus in the hepatic vein is seen in cirrhosis and malignancy because of an increased hepatic arterial supply and arteriovenous shunting. This technique has been shown to be a highly sensitive indicator of cirrhosis and metastases (44,45). Large prospective trials are presently underway to assess the predictive value of this technique for the presence of micrometastases in cancer patients before they can be detected by conventional imaging, and as a noninvasive means of diagnosing cirrhosis in chronic liver disease.

Another example of the use of transit studies is the detection of cardiopulmonary shunting. Echovist and agitated saline are too fragile to cross the normal pulmonary circulation but in the presence of pulmonary arteriovenous malformations (PAVMs) or a right to left cardiac shunt, systemic spectral Doppler signal is seen in the carotid artery after a peripheral venous injection (46). The signal changes can be quantified (in terms of the amount as well as presence of shunting) and can potentially replace the current radionuclide test.

Time intensity curves can be drawn for an area of interest to document microbubble transit through, for example, a tumor bed (47). The indices (e.g., bolus arrival time) derived from them can be used to construct true functional images by displaying them on a pixel-by-pixel basis as an overlay on the gray-scale image (Fig. 7). They are particularly promising for heterogeneous tissues such as tumors. These combined structural and functional maps hold great potential.

Table 2
Uses of Ultrasound Contrast Agents in Doppler Rescue Studies

1. Assessment of portal venous patency in cirrhosis (difficult because of increased liver attenuation of the ultrasound beam and/or weak venous signals due to slow flow)
2. Diagnosis of renal artery stenosis (difficult because of technical problems with deep abdominal vessels)
3. Tight carotid artery stenosis (to distinguish total occlusion from trickle flow)
4. TIPS shunts (often no signal can be obtained without contrast)
5. Transcranial Doppler (skull bone causes attenuation resulting in a high failure rate without contrast)

Active quantitation methods are based on the destruction of microbubbles and observation of the effects on contrast enhancement ("reperfusion kinetics"). Intermittent high power US pulses are used to destroy microbubbles within the beam and the rate of replenishment in the field can be used to calculate indices such as microcirculatory flow rate, a measure of tissue perfusion. Wei et al. (48) applied this principle to the measurement of myocardial blood flow in dogs by infusing microbubbles while scanning intermittently. They observed an exponential relationship between pulsing interval (PI) and video intensity (VI) [$VI = VI_{max(1-e^{\beta \cdot PI})}$ where VI_{max} is the maximal video intensity, seen at long pulsing intervals, and β is the constant describing the rate of rise of VI]. The initial upslope of this curve is proportional to microbubble speed as they refill the slice being insonated. A high-energy pulse of US can be administered to destroy the bubbles, and tissue refill is observed with nondestructive low acoustic power imaging to demonstrate tissue perfusion in real time. The rate of this refilling is a measure of regional tissue blood flow and has been used in the assessment of ischemic myocardium, and in renal transplants (49).

Liver-Specific Microbubbles

Microbubbles were initially thought to be solely blood pool agents but recently, some have been shown to have a hepatosplenic-specific parenchymal phase following disappearance from the blood pool (approximately three minutes after injection). Agents known to exhibit this late phase are Levovist (50), Sonavist (Schering, Germany) (51), and Sonazoid^{TM} (NC100100; Amersham, U.K.) (Table 1) (52). In this state, the bubbles are stationary, as shown by the absence of conventional Doppler signals. Their site of hepatic accumulation is unknown but may be within the reticuloendothelial system or they may simply pool in sinusoids. This late phase has a variable duration lasting under ~30 minutes with Levovist but longer with other agents such as Sonazoid and Sonavist. The tissue-specific phase can be imaged by bubble-specific modes such as loss of correlation (LOC) (50) and phase inversion (53).

Phase/Pulse Inversion Mode

The development of this novel mode was prompted by the desire to overcome the loss of spatial resolution of narrow band (dual frequency) harmonic imaging. Phase/pulse inversion mode (PIM) uses the full bandwidth of the transducer, which results in superior spatial resolution and higher contrast than harmonic gray scale or conventional color Doppler (53).

PIM detects nonlinear echoes from microbubbles (53). Liver malignancies appear as defects surrounded by an intensely bright parenchyma in the late liver-specific phase of microbubbles (Fig. 8). This technique has been shown to increase the sensitivity in the detection of focal liver malignancies by improving their conspicuity (54–56). In a multicenter study of 123 patients, the sensitivity to liver metastases increased from 71% to 88% and the mean size of detectable lesions improved by 50% to under one cm (57).

Loss of Correlation Mode and Applications

In this mode, also known as stimulated acoustic emission (SAE), microbubble disruption is seen as a transient strong signal in color or power Doppler. In loss of correlation mode (LOC), malignant liver tumors appear as defects surrounded by a color mosaic pattern when the liver is scanned some minutes after the administration of liver-specific agents. Blomley et al. (58) demonstrated that LOC improved the conspicuity of liver metastases and revealed new lesions not seen on conventional B-mode (Fig. 9). Subtle or isoechoic metastases could be demonstrated increasing the sensitivity of US to the detection of metastatic disease. In a further study of the specificity of LOC, a spectrum of benign and malignant focal liver lesions were assessed for LOC activity in the late phase of Levovist (59). Metastases and hepatocellular carcinoma (HCC) showed no or low LOC signals while hemangiomas and focal nodular hyperplasia (FNH) had significantly higher scores (Fig. 10).

However, LOC imaging has limitations. Its transient nature means that frames have to be reviewed in the cine loop (therefore not real time); the effect falls off at depths > 12 cm. It is very dependent on the position of the focal zone and its spatial resolution is that of color Doppler, two to four times worse than gray scale.

Recently developed LOC-based modes overcome some of these limitations; one such mode is ADI (Agent Detection Imaging; Siemens, California, U.S.) which exhibits better spatial filling since it is less focal zone dependent and has excellent spatial resolution (Fig. 10) (60).

Low Acoustic Power Real-Time Modes

Nondestructive real-time modes have largely replaced the disruptive methods in all applications in countries where SonoVue® is available. These low acoustic power bubble-specific modes such as power pulse inversion (Philips, Washington, U.S.) and the contrast pulse sequence (CPS) (Siemens, California, U.S.) minimize bubble destruction and have the added advantage of suppressing tissue harmonics (Fig. 11). These technological advances combined with the availability of more stable microbubbles (e.g., SonoVue, Bracco, Italy) have facilitated the development of real-time nondestructive [low mechanical index (MI)] imaging modes that can demonstrate the capillary bed as well as larger vessels. Contrast enhanced imaging of focal liver lesions may be divided into arterial (20–25 sec) and portal (45–90 sec) phases and real-time imaging allows these phases to be followed successively so that the dynamic enhancement pattern and vascular morphology may be assessed. Recent studies have shown that the vascular phase can improve the characterization of focal lesions such as hemangiomas which exhibit peripheral globular enhancement and centripetal filling-in, analogous to that seen on CT (Fig. 11) (60).

Contrast agents have been shown to be useful in improving the detection of HCCs, in differentiating HCC from regenerating nodules, and in detecting recurrence in treated lesions (Fig. 12). Two different approaches are used for this. Firstly, the hypervascularity of HCC can be exploited on arterial phase imaging to improve detection of small lesions (61,62). Secondly, most HCCs show as defects on late phase imaging with liver-specific agents, again improving their detection, while signal enhancement similar to surrounding parenchyma is seen within regenerating nodules (63).

Interventional US and Therapy

High Intensity Focused US

High intensity focused ultrasound (HIFU) as a therapeutic technique is not a new concept, but recent advances in probe design and alternate ultrasonic imaging methods make it likely to become a realistic clinical tool in the near future (64). The principle of HIFU is that a highly focused US beam is used to destroy a defined volume of tissue by inducing a rapid rise in temperature to greater than 50°C. Maintenance of this temperature for one to three seconds results in cell death—a single US exposure destroying a 0.5 ml volume of tissue. The surrounding tissue is not damaged. This noninvasive technique has been used to treat malignant tumors of the liver, prostate, and kidney and benign breast tumors via a percutaneous or transrectal approach without the need for general anesthesia (65,66). Although promising, HIFU is currently limited by the amount of tissue that can be destroyed by a single US exposure, the time required between exposures to allow local tissue cooling, the inability to treat through bone, and problems of monitoring therapy in real time. Technological advances promise to overcome many of these problems. Tissue ablated by HIFU is best observed using MR (66), which renders the treatment cumbersome and expensive. Since B-mode US does not distinguish between coagulated and normal tissue, alternate ultrasonic imaging methods such as elastography, reflex transmission imaging, and thermal imaging to depict the tissue damage are being explored (Fig. 13).

Future applications could include revascularization of the myocardium by the creation of channels in the ventricular wall (67) and the emergency treatment of internal hemorrhage by inducing hemostasis within bleeding vessels (68), for example, after trauma, biopsy, or catheterization. HIFU could also be deployed intraoperatively, e.g., in the treatment of liver metastases.

Ultrasound Drug and Gene Delivery

Intravascular US is known to enhance the effects of thrombolytic drugs. The addition of microbubbles further enhances thrombolytic activity by aiding penetration of the drug into the thrombus (69,70). Delivery to a thrombus can be accentuated by incorporating ligands on the surface of the microbubble that recognize receptors on the cell membrane; e.g., incorporation of a surface ligand that binds GPIIB/IIIA receptors on activated platelets (Fig. 14) (71).

US causes a transient increase in cell membrane permeability in a process known as sonoporation (Fig. 15). Using this technique, tissues can be targeted so that cellular uptake of a drug (e.g., a chemotherapeutic agent) or a gene is achieved (72). Sonoporation requires high acoustic powers (generally beyond those used for diagnosis but similar to those used in physiotherapy) but the power needed is markedly reduced when microbubbles are present. A drug or gene vector can be incorporated in or on the surface of the microbubbles and tracked in the circulation with an imaging beam, and when they are exposed to high power US, the microspheres rupture, releasing the agent in the vicinity of the target tissue (69,70). In the case of oncological drugs, this should have the advantage of decreasing the dose of the drug needed, so reducing systemic side effects. Encouraging initial in vitro studies have demonstrated sonoporation without inducing cell death (73). In another study, transfection of a reporter gene in a mouse heart increased 10-fold when a a microbubble carrying an adenovirus gene vector was used (74).

Interventional Procedures

There is a wide range of dedicated interventional transducers (i.e., intraoperative, laparoscopic, transrectal, Siterite^{TM}, etc. for intravenous access) which have broadened this field of application. Future endoscopic and laparoscopic US transducers will have built-in biopsy channels allowing both diagnostic biopsies and therapeutic applications (e.g., cryo-, RF-electrocautery, HIFU, microwave devices). Many transducers are already equipped with biopsy-guiding facilities and needle-tracking systems to enhance needle visualization (e.g., Ultraguide). Three-dimensional US may provide image information allowing multiplanar planning and execution of interventional procedures.

SUMMARY

US has undergone an impressive metamorphosis since its beginnings and now occupies a pivotal role at the forefront of radiological practice and research. Technological advances in electronics and computing have revolutionized US practice with ever expanding applications. Developments in transducer materials and array designs have resulted in greater bandwidths with improvements in spatial and contrast resolution. Developments in digital signal processing have produced innovations in beam forming and image display. Technological advances have resulted in novel imaging modes which exploit the nonlinear behavior of tissue and microbubble contrast agents. Microbubble contrast agents have dramatically extended the clinical and research applications of US. Novel nonlinear modes allow vessels down to the level of the microcirculation to be studied. Functional and quantitative studies allow interrogation of a wide spectrum of tissue beds. The advent of tissue-specific agents has improved the sensitivity and specificity of US in the detection and characterization of focal liver lesions. US has recently moved into therapeutic applications with HIFU and microbubble-assisted delivery of drugs and genes showing great promise. If the future of US echoes its past, its potential is boundless.

REFERENCES

1. Whittingham TA. New and future directions in ultrasonic imaging. Br J Radiol 1997; 70:S119–S132.
2. Whittingham TA. Modern developments in diagnostic ultrasound—Part 1: transducer and signal processing developments. Radiography 1995; 1:61–73.
3. Whittingham TA. Broadband transducers. Eur Radiol 1999; 9:S298–S303.
4. Foster FS. Transducer materials and probe construction. Ultrasound Med Biol 2000; 26(suppl 1):S2–S25.
5. Park SE, Shrout TR. Characteristics of relaxor based piezoelectric single crystals for ultrasonic transducers. IEEE Trans Ultrason Ferro Freq Contr 1998; 45:1071–1076.
6. Whittingham TA. An overview of digital technology in ultrasonic imaging. Eur Rad 1999; 9(suppl 3):S307–S311.
7. Entrekin RR, Porter BA, Sillesen HH, Wong AD, Cooperberg PL, Fix CH. Real-time spatial compound imaging: application to breast, vascular, and musculoskeletal ultrasound. Semin Ultrasound CT MR 2001; 22:50–64.
8. Cooperberg PL, Barberie J, Wong AD, Fix C. Extended field of view ultrasound. Semin Ultrasound CT MR 2001; 22:65–77.
9. Barberie J, Wong AD, Cooperberg PL, Carson BW. Extended field of view sonography in musculoskeletal disorders. Am J Roentgenol 1998; 171:751–757.
10. Lees WR. Ultrasound imaging in three and four dimensions. Semin Ultrasound CT MR 2001; 22:85–105.
11. Nelson TR. Three-dimensional imaging. Ultrasound Med Biol 2000; 26(suppl 1):S35–S38.
12. Johnson DD, Pretorius DH, Budorick NE, Jones MC, Lou KV, James GM, Nelson TR. Fetal lip and primary palate: three-dimensional versus two-dimensional US. Radiology 2000; 217:236–239.
13. Weismann CF, Forstner R, Prokop E, Rettenbacher T. Three-dimensional targeting: a new three-dimensional ultrasound technique to evaluate needle position during breast biopsy. Ultrasound Obstet Gynecol 2000; 16:359–364.
14. Desser TS, Jeffrey RB. Tissue harmonic imaging techniques: physical principles and clinical applications. Semin Ultrasound CT MR 2001; 22(suppl 1):1–10.
15. Whittingham TA. Tissue harmonic imaging. Eur Radiol 1999; 9(suppl 3):S323–S326.
16. Burns PN, Hope Simpson D, Averkiou MA. Nonlinear imaging. Ultrasound Med Biol 2000; 26(suppl 1):S19–S22.
17. Shapiro RS, Wagreich J, Parsons RB, Stancato-Pasik A, Yeh HC, Lao R. Tissue harmonic imaging sonography: evaluation of image quality compared with conventional sonography. Am J Roentgenol 1998; 171:1203–1206.
18. Desser TS, Jeffrey RB, Lane MJ. Tissue harmonic imaging: utility in abdominal and pelvic sonography. J Clin Ultrasound 1999; 27:135–142.
19. Hann LE, Bach AM, Cramer LD, Siegel D, Yoo HH, Garcia R. Hepatic sonography: comparison of tissue harmonic and standard sonography techniques. Am J Roentgenol 1999; 173:201–206.
20. Jang HJ, Lim HK, Lee WJ, Kim SH, Kim KA, Kim EY. Ultrasonographic evaluation of focal hepatic lesions: comparison of pulse inversion harmonic, tissue harmonic, and conventional imaging techniques. J Ultrasound Med 2000; 19:293–299.
21. Tanaka S, Oshikawa O, Kitamira T. Evaluation of tissue harmonic imaging in the diagnosis of liver tumors. Radiology 1998; 209(P):342.
22. Fuechsel FG, Bush NL, Bamber JC, Miller NR, Doyley MM, Cosgrove DO. An interactive display of freehand elasticity imaging (FEI) on breast masses in combination with ultrasound for improved understanding of breast pathology and better differential diagnosis. Radiology 2000; 217 (P):706.

23. Bamber JC. Ultrasound elasticity imaging: definition and technology. Eur Radiol 1999; 9(suppl 3):S327–S330.

24. Fatemi M, Greenleaf JF. Vibro-acoustography: an imaging modality based on ultra-sound-stimulated emission. Proc Natl Acad Sci USA 1999; 96:6603–6608.

25. Foster FS, Pavlin CJ, Harasiewicz KA, Christopher DA, Turnbull DH. Advances in ultrasound biomicroscopy. Ultrasound Med Biol 2000; 26:1–27.

26. Jones JP. Applications of acoustical microscopy in dermatology. In: Dunn F, ed. Ultra-sonic Tissue Characterization. New York: Springer-Verlag, 1996:201–212.

27. Saijo Y, Tanaka M, Okawai H, Dunn F. The ultrasonic properties of gastric cancer tis-sues obtained with a scanning acoustic microscope system. Ultrasound Med Biol 1991; 17:709–714.

28. Sasaki H, Saijo Y, Tanaka M, Okawai H, Terasawa Y, Yambe T, Nitta S. Influence of tissue preparation on the high frequency acoustic properties of normal kidney tissue. Ultrasound Med Biol 1996; 22:1261–1265.

29. Liu JB, Goldberg BB. 2-D and 3-D endoluminal ultrasound. Ultrasound Med Biol 2000; 26(suppl 1):S137–S139.

30. Krams R, Wentzel JJ, Oomen JA, Schuurbiers JC, Andhyiswara I, Kloet J, Post M, de Smet B, Borst C, Slager CJ, Serruys PW. Shear stress in atherosclerosis and vascular remodelling. Semin Interv Cardiol 1998; 3:39–44.

31. Cosgrove DO. Ultrasound contrast agents. In: Dawson P, Cosgrove DO, Grainger RG, eds. Textbook of Contrast Media. Oxford, U.K.: ISIS Medical Media, 1999:451–587.

32. Goldberg BB, Raichlen JS, Forsberg F, eds. Ultrasound Contrast Agents. 2nd ed. London: Martin Dunitz, 2001.

33. Harvey CJ, Blomley MJK, Eckersley RJ, Cosgrove DO. Developments in ultrasound contrast media. Eur Radiol 2001; 11:675–689.

34. de Jong N. Physics of microbubble scattering. In: Nanda N, Schlief R, Goldberg BB, eds. Advances in Echo Imaging Using Contrast Enhancement. 2d ed. Lancaster, England: Kluwer Academic, 1997:39–64.

35. Forsberg F, Shi WT. Physics of contrast microbubbles. In: Goldberg BB, Raichen JS, Forsberg F, eds. Ultrasound Contrast Agents. 2d ed. London: Martin Dunitz, 2001:15–24.

36. Albrecht T, Mattrey RF. Tumor imaging with ultrasound contrast. In: Thomsen HS, Muller RN, Mattrey RF, eds. Trends in Contrast Media Medical Radiology: Diagnostic Imaging and Radiation Oncology Series. Berlin: Springer, 1999:367–382.

37. Ayida G, Harris P, Kennedy PS, Seif M, Barlow D, Chamberlain P. Hysterosalpingo-contrast sonography (HyCoSy) using Echovist-200 in the outpatient investigation of infertility patients. Br J Radiol 1997; 69:910–913.

38. Darge K, Troeger J, Duetting T, Zieger B, Rohrschneider W, Moehring K, Weber C, Toenshoff B. Reflux in young patients: comparison of voiding US of the bladder and retrovesical space with echo enhancement versus voiding cystourethography for diagnosis. Radiology 1999; 210:201–207.

39. Claudon M, Plouin PF, Baxter GM, Rohban T, Devos DM. Renal arteries in patients at risk of renal artery stenosis: multicenter evaluation of the echo-enhancer SH U 508A at color and spectral Doppler US. Radiology 2000; 214:739–746.

40. Mulvagh SL, DeMaria AN, Feinstein SB, Burns PN, Kaul S, Miller JG, Monaghan M, Porter TR, Shaw LJ, Villanueva FS. Contrast echocardiography: current and future applications. J Am Soc Echocardiogr 2000; 13:331–342.

41. Cheng SC, Dy TC, Feinstein SB. Contrast echocardiography: review and future direc-tions. Am J Cardiol 1998; 81(12A):41G–48G.

42. Cwaig J, Xie F, O'Leary E, Kricsfeld D, Dittrich H, Porter TR. Detection of angiographically significant coronary artery disease with accelerated intermittent imaging after intravenous administration of ultrasound contrast material. Am Heart J 2000; 139:675–683.

43. Blomley MJK, Eckersley RJ, Cosgrove DO. Potential for quantitation. In: Thomsen HS, Muller RN, Mattrey RF, eds. Trends in Contrast Media. Medical Radiology: Diagnostic Imaging and Radiation Oncology Series. Berlin: Springer, 1999:343–353.

44. Blomley MJK, Lim ALP, Harvey CJ, Patel N, Eckersley RJ, Basilico R, Heckemann R, Butler-Barnes J, Urbank A, Cosgrove DO, Taylor-Robinson SD. Liver microbubble transit time compared with histology in diffuse liver disease: a cross sectional study. Gut 2003; 52:1188–1193.

45. Blomley MJ, Albrecht T, Cosgrove DO, Jayaram V, Eckersley RJ, Patel N, Taylor-Robinson S, Bauer A, Schlief R. Liver vascular transit time analyzed with dynamic hepatic venography with bolus injections of an US contrast agent: early experience in 7 patients with metastases. Radiology 1998; 209:862–866.

46. Blomley MJK, Harvey CJ, Hughes JM, Heckemann R, Eckersley R, Cosgrove DO. Can relative signal changes in the intensity of systemic spectral Doppler signals after bolus injections of microbubbles measure pulmonary AV shunting noninvasively? Radiology 1999; 213(P):1145.

47. Albrecht T, Patel N, Cosgrove DO, Jayaram V, Blomley M. Breast masses studied with the ultrasound contrast agent EchoGen. Acad Radiol 1998; 5(suppl 1):S195–S198.

48. Wei K, Jayaweera AR, Firoozan S, Linka A, Skyba DM, Kaul S. Quantification of myocardial blood flow with ultrasound induced destruction of microbubbles administered as a constant venous infusion. Circulation 1998; 97:473–483.

49. Harvey CJ, Lynch M, Blomley MJK, Cosgrove DO, Warrens A. Quantitation of real-time perfusion with the microbubble optison using power pulse inversion mode in renal transplants. Eur Radiol 2001; 11(suppl 1): 103.

50. Blomley MJK, Albrecht T, Cosgrove DO, Jayaram V, Butler-Barnes J. Stimulated acoustic emission in the liver parenchyma with the ultrasound contrast agent Levovist. Lancet 1998; 351:568.

51. Forsberg F, Goldberg BB, Liu JB, Merton DA, Rawool NM, Shi WT. Tissue-specific US contrast agent for evaluation of hepatic and splenic parenchyma. Radiology 1999; 210:125–132.

52. Leen E, Ramnarine K, Kyriakopoulou K, Gordon PB, Mc Dicken WN, Mc Ardle C. Improved characterization of focal liver tumors: dynamic Doppler imaging using NC100100: a new liver-specific echo-enhancer. Radiology 1998; 209(P):293.

53. Hope Simpson D, Chin CT, Burns PN. Pulse inversion Doppler: a new method for detecting nonlinear echoes from microbubble contrast agents. IEEE Trans Ultrason Ferroelectr Freq Contr 1999; 46:372–382.

54. Harvey CJ, Blomley MJ, Eckersley RJ, Cosgrove DO, Patel N, Heckemann RA, Butler-Barnes J. Hepatic malignancies: improved detection with pulse-inversion US in late phase of enhancement with SH U 508A-early experience. Radiology 2000; 216:903–908.

55. Harvey CJ, Blomley MJ, Eckersley RJ, Heckemann RA, Butler-Barnes J, Cosgrove DO. Pulse inversion mode imaging of liver specific microbubbles: improved detection of sub-centimetre metastases. Lancet 2000; 355:807–808.

56. Albrecht T, Hoffmann CW, Schmitz SA, Schettler S, Overberg A, Germer CT, Wolf KJ. Phase inversion sonography during the liver specific phase of Levovist: improved detection of liver metastases. Am J Roentgenol 2001; 176:1191–1198.

57. Albrecht T, Blomley MJ, Burns PN, Wilson S, Harvey CJ, Leen E, Claudon M, Calliada F, Correas JM, LaFortune M, Campani R, Hoffmann CW, Cosgrove DO, LeFevre F. Improved detection of hepatic metastases with pulse inversion ultrasonography during the liver-specific phase of SHU 508A (levovist): a multicenter study. Radiology 2003; 227:361–370.

58. Blomley MJ, Albrecht T, Cosgrove DO, Patel N, Jayaram V, Butler-Barnes J, Eckersley RJ, Bauer A, Schlief R. Improved imaging of liver metastases with stimulated acoustic emission

in the late phase of enhancement with the US contrast agent SH U 508A: early experience. Radiology 1999; 210:409–416.

59. Blomley MJ, Sidhu PS, Cosgrove DO, Albrecht T, Harvey CJ, Heckemann RA, Butler-Barnes J, Eckersley RJ, Basilico R. Do different types of liver lesions differ in their uptake of the microbubble SH U 508A in its late liver phase: early experience. Radiology 2001; 220:661–667.

60. Bryant TH, Blomley MJ, Albrecht T, Sidhu PS, Leen EL, Basilico R, Pilcher JM, Bushby LH, Hoffman CW, Harvey CJ, Lynch M, Mac Quarrie J, Paul D, Cosgrove DO. Liver phase uptake of a liver-specific microbubble improves characterization of liver lesions: a prospective multi-center study. Radiology 2004; 232:799–809.

61. Wilson SR, Burns PN, Muradali D, Wilson JA, Lai X. Harmonic hepatic US with microbubble contrast agent: Initial experience showing improved characterization of hemangioma, hepatocellular carcinoma and metastasis. Radiology 2000; 215:153–161.

62. Choi BI, Kim TK, Han JK, Kim AY, Seong CK, Park SJ. Vascularity of hepatocellular carcinoma: assessment with contrast-enhanced second harmonic versus conventional power Doppler US. Radiology 2000; 214:167–172.

63. Blomley M, Cosgrove DO, Sidhu P, Albrecht T, Heckemann R, Butler-Barnes J, Eckersley R. Does stimulated acoustic emission (SAE) imaging with the US contrast agent Levovist improve specificity in imaging focal liver lesions with US? Eur Radiol 1999; 9;(suppl 1):S64.

64. ter Haar GR. Intervention and therapy. Ultrasound Med Biol 2000; 26(suppl 1):S51–S54.

65. Visioli AG, Rivens IH, ter Haar GR, Horwich A, Huddart RA, Moskovic E, Padhani A, Glees J. Preliminary results of a phase I dose escalation clinical trial using focused ultrasound in the treatment of localised tumours. Eur J Ultrasound 1999; 9:11–18.

66. Hynynen K, Freund WR, Cline HE, Chung AH, Watkins RD, Vetro JP, Jolesz FA. A clinical noninvasive, MR imaging monitored ultrasound surgery method. Radiographics 1996; 16:185–195.

67. Smith NB, Hynynen K. The feasibility of using focused ultrasound for transmyocardial revascularisation. Ultrasound Med Biol 1998; 24:1045–1054.

68. Martin RW, Vaezy S, Kaczkowski P, Keilman G, Carter S, Caps M, Beach K, Plett M, Crum L. Hemostasis of punctured vessels using Doppler-guided high intensity focused ultrasound. Ultrasound Med Biol 1999; 25:985–990.

69. Unger EC. Targeting and delivery of drugs with contrast agents. In: Thomsen HS, Muller RN, Mattrey RF, eds. Trends in Contrast Media. Medical Radiology: Diagnostic Imaging and Radiation Oncology Series. Berlin: Springer, 1999:405–412.

70. Miller MW. Gene transfection and drug delivery. Ultrasound Med Biol 2000; 26(suppl 1):S59–S62.

71. Wu Y, Unger EC, McCreery TP, Sweitzer RH, Shen D, Wu G, Vielhauer MD. Binding and lysing of blood clots using MRX-408. Invest Radiol 1998; 33:880–885.

72. Miller DL, Bao S, Gies RA, Thrall BD. Ultrasonic enhancement of gene transfection in murine melanoma cells. Ultrasound Med Biol 1999; 25:1425–1430.

73. Brayman AA, Coppage ML, Vaidya S, Miller MW. Transient poration and cell surface receptor removal from human lymphocytes in vitro by 1 MHz ultrasound. Ultrasound Med Biol 1999; 25:999–1008.

74. Shohet RV, Chen S, Zhou YT, Wang Z, Meidell RS, Unger RH, Grayburn PA. Echocardiographic destruction of albumin microbubbles directs gene delivery to the myocardium. Circulation 2000; 101:2554–2556.

75. Harvey CJ, Pilcher JM, Eckersley RJ, Blomley MJ, Cosgrove DO. Advances in ultrasound. Clin Radiol 2002; 57:157–177.

76. Blomley MJ, Cooke JC, Unger EC, Monaghan MJ, Cosgrove DO. Microbubble contrast agents: new era in ultrasound. BMJ 2001; 322:1222–1225.

11

Ultrasound Competency

William Lunn
Interventional Pulmonary, Baylor College of Medicine, Houston, Texas, U.S.A.

Armin Ernst
Beth Israel Deaconess Medical Center, Boston, Massachusetts, U.S.A.

INTRODUCTION

Ultrasound (US) was born of tragedy. With the sinking of the *Titanic* in 1912, scientists around the world became interested in developing technology that would allow vessels to locate and avoid icebergs and other maritime impediments. Intense research led to the development of sound assisted navigation and ranging (SONAR) which employed sound waves to detect and map the location of underwater obstacles. As scientists learned more about the ability of sound waves to detect and map structures in the sea, the idea surfaced that this technology could also be applied to the human body for medical purposes. The first paper on medical US was presented by Dr. Dussik of Austria in the late 1940s (1). Pulsed Doppler applications were developed in the mid-1970s which resulted in the introduction of vascular US. Technology has continued to progress at a rapid pace allowing for the development of more compact probes, higher resolution images, and software to create 3-dimensional imagery.

Medical and surgical specialists alike have embraced US in clinical practice, finding it to be indispensable for diagnostic purposes and for facilitation of invasive procedures. Compact US machines have become ubiquitous in hospital and outpatient clinics. As physicians' utilization of US has increased dramatically, the question as to what constitutes the physicians' competence to perform and interpret US examinations has arisen. The purpose of this chapter is to review the concept of medical competence, explore the controversy surrounding US credentialing, and discuss the existing criteria for US training and credentialing.

COMPETENCE DEFINED

The concept of medical competence is a difficult one to define. When one seeks a definition of competence from traditional dictionaries, one is confronted with information that is not applicable to the medical field. For example, The Merriam-Webster Dictionary offers several definitions of competence including "a sufficiency of means for the necessities of life," "the quality or state of being competent," and "the knowledge that enables a person to speak and understand a language" (2). The Institute for International Medical Education (IIME) has compiled an online dictionary to address the need for definitions of terms more applicable to physicians (3). The IIME offers an elegant and thoughtful definition of competence as follows:

> Possession of a satisfactory level of relevant knowledge and acquisition of a range of relevant skills that include interpersonal and technical components at a certain point in the educational process. Such knowledge and skills are necessary to perform the tasks that reflect the scope of professional practices. Competence may differ from 'performance,' which denotes actions taken in a real life situation. Competence is therefore not the same as 'knowing.' On the contrary, it may well be about recognizing one's own limits. The more experienced the professional being tested, the more difficult it is to create a tool to assess their actual understandings, abilities and the complex skills of the tasks they undertake. A holistic integration of understandings, abilities and professional judgments, i.e., a 'generic' model, is one where competence is not necessarily directly observable, but rather can be inferred from performance.

Physician organizations, in an attempt to encourage members to acquire and maintain necessary knowledge and skills to function at peak, have developed models of competence that usually involve three broad categories: (i) acquisition of continuing medical education (CME), (ii) peer review, and (iii) performance appraisal by periodic examination. The American Board of Internal Medicine (ABIM), for example, now requires members who are board-certified specialists who wish to re-certify to complete a three-step process of re-certification which is to take place at least every ten years. Thus, there is a general consensus that competence involves knowledge, skills, and an ability to employ both successfully in practice.

ULTRASOUND COMPETENCE

As physicians from several specialties have participated in the current renaissance of US, much controversy surrounds the question of as to which specialty does US belong. Is US the exclusive purview of radiology, or must other disciplines also hold sway? In 1999, recognizing the explosion of US use among physicians, the American Medical Association

House of Delegates passed Resolution 802, which affirmed that US is within the scope of practice of appropriately trained nonradiologists and called for each specialty to develop a set of criteria to define the appropriate training required for specialists to employ the technology with skill and accuracy (4).

The American College of Radiology (ACR), which had developed a practice for performing and interpreting diagnostic US examinations in 1992, responded by revising their guideline in 2000 (5). The ACR guideline states that physicians performing and/or interpreting diagnostic US should meet one of three criteria: (i) certification in Radiology or Diagnostic Radiology by an American or Canadian board of radiology and performance and interpretation of 300 US examinations in the last 36 months; (ii) completion of an accredited diagnostic radiology residency program and performance and interpretation of 500 US examinations in the last 36 months; (iii) completion of an accredited residency program in the specialty practiced by the physician, 200 hours of Category I CME credit in the subspecialty in which US reading occurs, and 500 US cases interpreted with supervision during the past 36 months.

Surgical and medical specialists regarded these criteria as too restrictive and many set out to devise their own standards of competence for the purposes of credentialing. Nonradiologists began looking for models by which they might develop criteria unique to the use of US in their area of interest. The Task Force on Clinical Competence (TFCC), a multidisciplinary organization formed in 1998 by the American College of Cardiology (ACC), the American Heart Association (AHA), the American College of Physicians (ACP), and the American Society of Internal Medicine (ASIM), serves as such a model. The TFCC was charged with the responsibility of devising competency criteria for physicians wishing to perform certain cardiovascular procedures, including echocardiography. The TFCC guideline for credentialing for echocardiography was published in 2003 and remains one of the most comprehensive and well-reasoned documents of its kind (6).

The TFCC identified four areas that must be mastered in order to be competent in adult echocardiography: (i) basic knowledge of US physics, (ii) technical aspects of the examination, (iii) knowledge of cardiac anatomy and physiology, and (iv) recognition of simple and complex pathology. Moreover, the TFCC recognized that different specialists may require or seek different levels of expertise with echocardiography. Therefore, three different levels of training were proposed in order to define various levels of competency. Level 1 training, which should have a duration of at least three months, includes mastery of the cognitive skills outlined above, the performance of 75 echocardiograms, and the interpretation of 150 examinations. The performance and interpretation of examinations must be supervised by a competent person in the field. The intent of Level 1 training is to make the physician a competent screener for disease who still requires support from and consultation with an expert. Level 2 training, which should have a duration of at least six months, includes the above coginitive skills to be mastered plus the performance of 150 examinations and the interpretation of 300 examinations. The intent is to make the physician an independent echo-cardiographer. Level 3 training, which should have duration of at least 12 months, includes the above mentioned skills that must be mastered plus the performance of 300 examinations and the interpretation of 750 examinations. The purpose of level 3 training is to provide the physician with a level of expertise high enough to permit the physician to serve as a director of an echocardiography laboratory.

Physicians may seek to prove their competence by taking and passing the Examination of Special Competence in Adult Echocardiography (ASCeXAM), the written board of the National Board of Echocardiography (NBE). While the board examination is not mandatory for credentialing purposes, it is essential in order to be certified by the NBE and represents a high level of achievement in the field. Finally, in order to maintain competence, the TFCC recommends that physicians with level 1 or level 2 training perform and/or interpret a minimum of 300 echocardiograms per year, while physicians with level 3 training should perform 500 examinations per year.

The American Registry of Diagnostic Medical Sonographers (ARDMS) serves as another model for US credentialing. The ARDMS was incorporated in 1975 and is a nonprofit organization that creates credentialing guidelines and administers examinations to physicians and medical sonographers. The ARDMS awards credentials in diagnostic medical sonography, cardiac sonography, and vascular sonography. There are discreet physician pathways in ARMDS certification. Physicians are required to demonstrate formal education (i.e., residency or fellowship) or informal education (i.e., CME) in US training including the performance of US examinations. Physicians sitting for the board examination in diagnostic sonography must pass a two-part exam with questions on US physics and abdominal sonography.

The American Institute for US in Medicine (AIUM), formed in 1952 to promote the appropriate use of the technology in medicine, also provides a guideline for physician credentialing. The AIUM first developed a guideline for physicians performing and interpreting US examinations in 1993 and the latest revision was approved in September 2003 (7). According to the 2003 guideline, physicians performing and/or interpreting diagnostic US should meet one of the following criteria: (i) completion of a residency, fellowship, or postgraduate training that includes at least three months of supervised US training and involvement in performing and interpreting at least 300 examinations, or (ii) in the absence of formal training, the physician must have completed 100 hours of Category I CME dedicated to diagnostic US and must have been involved with the performance and interpretation of 300 examinations in a three-year period and in a supervised setting.

US Competence: New Guidelines for Nonradiologists

Nonradiologists have contended that the above guidelines are not appropriate for their specialties because the number of supervised examinations required for training is excessive and that the amount of formal training or CME hours is also excessive for the types of focused examinations that they perform. Experts argued that fast track courses could be devised to quickly credential specialists, to perform US on organ systems in which they have already demonstrated expertise. However, there has been a great deal of debate in the literature in which nonradiologists have defended the concept of fast track training while radiologists have countered that lowering the requirements for training may lead to medical errors and adversely affect the patients (8–11).

Many medical and surgical specialties that employ US in practice, acknowledging the 1999 AMA resolution, have identified the need to create a comprehensive set of training and credentialing guidelines, but few have done so. One of the first groups to devise new training and credentialing criteria was the American College of Emergency Physicians (ACEP). The ACEP guidelines were based upon the initial recommendations made by the Society for Academic Emergency Medicine (SAEM) in 1994 (12). The SAEM recommendations were centered on the concept, previously outlined, that physicians performing US require both cognitive and practical skills. Therefore, the SAEM recommended that 40 hours of instruction should be taken in emergency US, followed by the performance of 150 supervised examinations. No certifying exam was proposed and no requirement for maintenance of competency was detailed.

In 2001, the ACEP detailed slightly different training and credentialing criteria (13). The ACEP identified residency-based and postgraduate US training as pathways for attaining competency in emergency US. While the residency-based criteria did not specify a minimum number of hours of education dedicated to cognitive training, the postgraduate pathway mandated at least 16 hours of cognitive instruction followed by the performance of 150 supervised US examinations. The ACEP statement also mandated that physicians obtain CME in US periodically after training in order to maintain competency, but the guideline did not specify the number of hours of CME or the timeframe in which they must be earned. Thus, when comparing the SAEM guidelines to that of the ACEP, the ACEP required less time in cognitive training, the same amount of practical experience, and dedication to further learning in order to maintain competency. Neither organization offered a standardized board examination in emergency ultrasonography.

The American Society of Diagnostic and Interventional Nephrology (ASDIN) (14) devised training and credentialing criteria for US of the bladder and kidneys in 2002. The current ASDIN guidelines identify fellowship-based and postgraduate training pathways. Physicians in fellowship are required to devote six weeks to US training. Physicians who have completed their fellowships are required to complete 50 hours of CME training as follows: three hours in basics of US physics, four hours of basic US interpretation, and 43 hours in the performance and interpretation of US examinations of the kidney and bladder. A total of 125 studies must be completed and 80 of these must be under direct supervision. The ASDIN certifies appropriate candidates meeting the above criteria for a period of five years. Re-certification may be obtained by performing 100 studies per year, providing documentation of accuracy of the interpretation for 40 studies or 10% of all studies performed, and earning 30 hours of CME every three years with a minimum of five hours devoted to ultrasonography. No standardized examination is offered for ASDIN certification or re-certification.

The American Society of Breast Surgeons (ASBS) (15) developed a breast US certification program for surgeons in 2002 that consisted of demonstrating cognitive and practical skills and passing a standardized written examination. The current ASBS guidelines require that physicians meet the following criteria: (i) current certification by the American Board of Surgery, (ii) a minimum of one year of experience in the performance and interpretation of breast US, (iii) documentation of a minimum of 100 breast US examinations per year, 80 diagnostic, and 20 interventional examinations, (iv) a minimum of 15 hours of CME in breast US. The written exams are currently offered twice a year to qualified candidates and consist of approximately 100 multiple choice questions covering all aspects of breast ultrasonography. Surgeons who satisfy the above criteria and pass the written exam are certified by the ASBS.

Though many specialties have yet to create US training and credentialing criteria, there remains a tremendous physician interest in obtaining US proficiency. It is interesting to note that there are currently 16 one-year fellowships in emergency medicine US offered in the United States. Moreover, a number of mini-fellowships and one-to-two day training courses are also offered each year in areas such as thyroid US, focused abdominal US, limited obstetrical US, renal US, and thoracic US.

CONCLUSIONS

US has become an integral part of the practice of many medical and surgical specialists over the last 15 years. AMA House Resolution 802, while acknowledging the right of nonradiologists to perform and interpret US examinations, has challenged the physician community to develop thoughtful standards by which training and credentialing may take place. Additionally, some third party players have begun to link training credentials of nonradiologists to US reimbursement. Some specialties have answered the AMA's call by developing and continuously improving training standards while others, such as the pulmonary and critical care community, are yet to respond. It is our hope that physicians will compel their medical societies to develop appropriate criteria to assure that physicians are employing US with judgment and skill to the benefit of their patients.

REFERENCES

1. Newman PG, Rozycki GS. The history of ultrasound. Surg Clin North Am 1998; 78(suppl 2):179–195.
2. Merriam-Webster's Collegiate Dictionary. 11th ed. Springfield, MA: Merriam-Webster Publisher, 2003.
3. www.iime.org/glossary.htm.
4. American Medical Association House of Delegates. H-230.960. Privileging for ultrasound imaging. 802.99.2001.
5. American College of Radiology. ACR practice guideline for performing and interpreting diagnostic ultrasound examinations. In: Practice Guidelines. Reston, VA: American College of Radiology, 2000:573–575.
6. Quinones MA, Douglas PS, Foster E, Gorcsan J III, Lewis JF, Pearlman AS, Rychik J, Salcedo EE, Seward JB, Stevenson JG, et al. ACC/AHA clinical competence statement on echocardiography. J Am Coll Cardiol 2003; 41(suppl 4):687–708.
7. American Institute for Ultrasound in Medicine. Official statement: training guidelines for physicians who evaluate and interpret diagnostic ultrasound examinations. Laurel, MD: AIUM, 2003.
8. Rozycki GS, Shackford SR. Ultrasound: what every trauma surgeon should know. J Trauma 1996; 40:1–4.
9. Connor PD, Deutchman ME, Hahn RG. Training in obstetric sonography in family medicine residency programs: results of a nationwide survey and suggestions for a teaching strategy. J Am Board Fam Pract 1994; 7:124–129.
10. Heller M. Emergency ultrasound: out of the acoustic shadows. Ann Emerg Med 1997; 29:380–382.
11. Hertzberg BS, Kliewer MA, Bowie JD, Carroll BA, DeLong DH, Gray L, Nelson RC. Physician training requirements in sonography: how many cases are needed for competence? Am J Roentgenol 2000; 174:1221–1227.
12. Mateer J, Plummer D, Heller M, Olson D, Jehle D, Overton D, Gussow L. Model curriculum for physician training in emergency ultrasonography. Ann Emerg Med 1994; 23:95–102.
13. American College of Emergency Medicine Emergency Ultrasound Guidelines. Ann Emerg Med 2001; 38(suppl 4):470–481.
14. American Society of Diagnostic and Interventional Nephrology Guidelines for Training in Renal Sonography. Semin Dial 2002; 15(suppl 6):442–444.
15. American Society of Breast Surgeons. Guidelines for Certification in Breast Ultrasonography, 2002.

Index